Practical Procedures in Nephrology

Practical Procedures in Nephrology

Edited by

Laurence R I Baker MA MD FRCP FRCPE

Consultant Physician and Nephrologist, Directorate of Renal Medicine and
Transplantation, St Bartholomew's Hospital, London, United Kingdom

Martin J Hurst BSc MB MRCP(UK)

Formerly Consultant Nephrologist, Directorate of Renal Medicine and
Transplantation, St Bartholomew's Hospital, London, United Kingdom

Christopher J Rudge FRCS

Consultant Transplant Surgeon, Directorate of Renal Medicine and
Transplantation, Royal London Hospital, London, United Kingdom

Mohammed S Sobeh FRCS

Consultant in General, Vascular and Transplant Surgery, Department of
Vascular Surgery, Royal London Hospital, London, United Kingdom

A member of the Hodder Headline Group
LONDON
Co-published in the USA by Oxford University Press, Inc., New York

First published in Great Britain in 2000 by
Arnold, a member of the Hodder Headline Group,
338 Euston Road, London NW1 3BH

http://www.arnoldpublishers.com

Co-published in the USA by
Oxford University Press Inc.,
198 Madison Avenue, New York, NY 10016
Oxford is a registered trademark of Oxford University Press

Whilst the advice and information in this book are believed to be true and accurate
at the date of going to press, neither the authors nor the publisher can accept
any legal responsibility or liability for any errors or omissions that may be made.
In particular (but without limiting the generality of the preceding disclaimer) every
effort has been made to check drug dosages; however, it is still possible that errors
have been missed. Furthermore, dosage schedules are constantly being revised
and new side-effects recognized. For these reasons the reader is strongly urged
to consult the drug companies' printed instructions before administering any of
the drugs recommended in this book.

British Library Cataloguing in Publication Data
A catalogue record for this book is available from the British Library

Library of Congress Cataloging-in-Publication Data
A catalog record for this book is available from the Library of Congress

ISBN 0 340 74083 3

1 2 3 4 5 6 7 8 9 10

Publisher: Georgina Bentliff
Production Editor: Wendy Rooke
Production Controller: Priya Gohil

Typeset in 10/13 pt Sabon by Scribe Design, Gillingham, Kent
Printed and bound in India by Ajanta Offset & Packagings Ltd, New Delhi

What do you think about this book? Or any other Arnold title?
Please send your comments to feedback.arnold@hodder.co.uk

CONTENTS

PREFACE

This text is aimed mainly at those who will carry out common practical procedures in patients with renal disease, particularly those with acute and chronic renal failure. Our hope is that it will be of value to trainees in nephrology and transplant and access surgery, and that it will be a source of reference to those about to begin or those who are already engaged in the treatment of patients with renal disease.

In general, we have considered procedures in a structured manner as follows:

1 Introduction (including indications and contraindications)
2 Pre-procedure assessment
3 Equipment required
4 Positioning of the patient
5 Anaesthesia
6 The procedure itself
7 Post-procedure management and care
8 Complications and their management.

We emphasize that, with the exception of removal of temporary venous and arterial access devices and temporary (hard) peritoneal catheters, all the procedures described in Chapters 2–5 inclusive require written, informed consent from the patient.

The procedures here described will need to be explained carefully to the patient in every case. We have not, in general, included an account of such counselling and obtaining of consent when describing procedures in individual chapters.

We have not attempted a comprehensive text encompassing all practical aspects of the investigation and management of patients with renal disease. Some items, such as the technique of urine microscopy, have been omitted as we feel they are the province of all medical practitioners rather than being exclusive to practitioners of renal medicine and surgery. Some, such as the renal transplant operation and transplant nephrectomy, have been omitted because they are the province of more senior staff. Still others, such as percutaneous nephrostomy, needle aspiration of a renal cyst, renal arteriography, angioplasty and stent insertion, are omitted because we feel them to be the province of the radiologist and urologist.

In several instances, more than one technique may be employed. Again, we have not attempted a comprehensive account of each and every alternative. Rather, we describe here methods that are widely employed and that we have ourselves found to be effective.

Omissions notwithstanding, we hope this text will be of interest and assistance to those working in renal and transplant units who must carry out the procedures we describe on a regular basis.

We thank Mr Sadiq Ahmed, Dr Alistair Chesser, Dr Simon Fletcher, Mr Islam Junaid, Professor Hartmut Malluche, Dr David New and Dr Judith Webb for helpful advice, Mrs Julie Jessop for secretarial assistance, Mrs Jennifer Fox and Ms Ann Stratham for production of the photographs and line drawings, respectively, and the Trustees of St Bartholomew's Hospital for financial assistance. Most of all, we thank Dr Peter Altman and Ms Georgina Bentliff for editorial assistance and encouragement.

chapter 1

VENEPUNCTURES AND CANNULATIONS

PRESERVING VESSELS FOR HAEMODIALYSIS ACCESS

Too many venepunctures are carried out upon patients with renal disease. Precious veins needed for fashioning of arteriovenous fistulae are frequently damaged or rendered useless for this purpose by venepuncture or cannulation for intravenous infusion. The most precious veins are the forearm cephalic, antecubital and upper arm cephalic veins (Figure 1.1), particularly those of the non-dominant arm where it is most desirable to fashion an arteriovenous fistula.

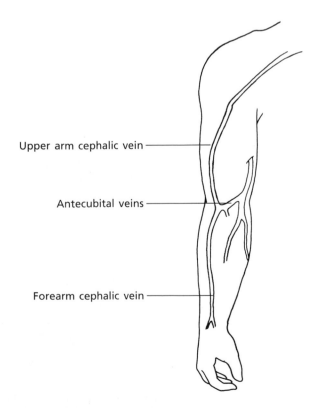

Upper arm cephalic vein

Antecubital veins

Forearm cephalic vein

Figure 1.1 Preferred veins for haemodialysis access.

Venepuncture and cannulation in these patients should be, whenever possible, restricted to the dorsum of the hand, the anterior aspect of the forearm and, occasionally, the feet.

The first consideration is to ask oneself whether blood sampling is really necessary. Daily checks on serum chemistry are often requested as a routine in patients with renal impairment, whereas less frequent investigation would be sufficient. Sometimes, the laboratory already have a specimen of blood or serum which could be used for the investigation in hand without further venepuncture. Sometimes a blood sample obtained by finger or thumb prick rather than by venepuncture will suffice, as in the case of blood glucose or haematocrit estimation. In patients already established on haemodialysis, blood samples can be obtained pre-dialysis from the access site which must in any event be used.

Diabetic patients present especial difficulty in respect of vascular access surgery owing to the increased prevalence of vascular disease in this group of patients. Quite often, it will be impossible to fashion a satisfactory forearm arteriovenous fistula in a diabetic with renal failure. The larger brachial artery will need to be employed. Antecubital veins are thus particularly precious in diabetics.

If the patient already has an arteriovenous fistula, this should not be cannulated for blood sampling or attempted intravenous infusion. Blood samples are often taken by phlebotomists who are not medically qualified and venous access for infusion established by very junior doctors. One way of avoiding error in this area is illustrated in Figure 1.2. More conventional approaches include the use of patient arm bands and documentation in case notes and above the patient's bed.

If intravenous administration of fluid or drugs is necessary, forearm and antecubital veins should be avoided in patients who may in the future require

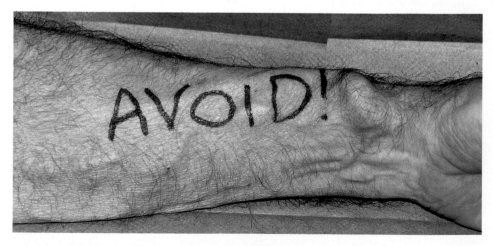

Figure 1.2 Protection of an arteriovenous fistula. Reprinted with permission from Kumar P, Clark ML (eds) *Clinical Medicine*, 4th edn, 1998.

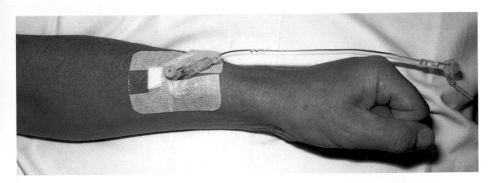

Figure 1.3 Intravenous infusion set up in exactly the wrong place in a right-handed patient with chronic renal failure who will later need a left (non-dominant) arm radiocephalic fistula. Reprinted with permission from Kumar P, Clark ML (eds) *Clinical Medicine*, 4th edn, 1998.

fashioning of an arteriovenous fistula, even if this requires insertion of a jugular venous cannula. Administration of agents which may cause chemical phlebitis is a particular danger in renal patients. If an antibacterial agent such as erythromycin or dextrose in concentrations between 10 and 50 per cent must be administered intravenously, peripheral veins of the arm – particularly the cephalic and antecubital veins – should be avoided and the jugular route employed.

Cardiac disease is common in renal patients and angiography, particularly coronary angiography, is frequently necessary. Two means of arterial access are available to the cardiologist, namely a cut-down on the brachial artery and percutaneous access via the femoral artery. The nephrologist should encourage his or her cardiologist colleague to use the latter route to avoid damaging the brachial artery, which may be required later for fashioning of a brachial fistula.

An intravenous infusion set up in exactly the wrong place in a right-handed patient who will later require a left forearm arteriovenous fistula is illustrated in Figure 1.3.

Patients established on regular dialysis may require admission to an intensive care unit owing to an intercurrent illness, and some patients admitted to intensive care with acute renal failure do not recover renal function and subsequently require renal replacement therapy. The nephrologist should defend radial and brachial arteries as well as cephalic and antecubital veins of such patients against cannulation if at all possible. Above all, patients and staff should be made aware of the need to protect the relevant veins and, if present, arteriovenous fistulae.

INTRAMUSCULAR INJECTIONS

These should be avoided if at all possible in patients who are anticoagulated long term or who receive intermittent anticoagulation with heparin during haemodialysis sessions owing to the risk of haematoma formation.

CANNULATION OF ARTERIOVENOUS FISTULAE

Introduction
Typically this is carried out by nurses to provide vascular access for haemodialysis. Fistulae should not be cannulated for any other reason, except in an emergency.

Pre-procedure assessment
Two access sites should be identified (or one if single-needle dialysis is contemplated); time spent on reconnaissance is never wasted. The arteriovenous anastomosis site should be identified and avoided. The antecubital fossa should also be avoided, if possible, for it is uncomfortable for the patient to maintain the arm straight during several hours of treatment by haemodialysis. 'Universal' precautions, which include the use of protective goggles, gowns and gloves, should, as the term implies, be employed in every case and not restricted to patients known to be potentially infectious, such as those who are hepatitis B surface antigen, hepatitis C antibody or HIV antibody positive.

Equipment
See Figure 1.4.

Positioning of patient
The patient should lie supine, recline at 45 degrees or sit in an armchair in a warm environment with the arm in a comfortable position.

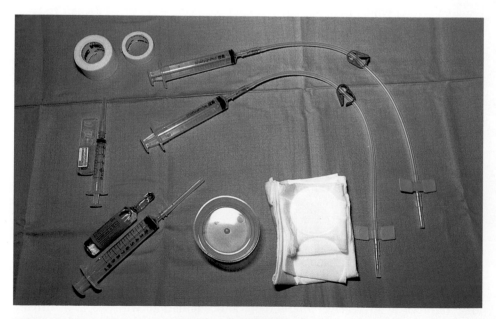

Figure 1.4 Trolley laid up for cannulation of arteriovenous fistula.

Anaesthesia

In many patients, the skin at venepuncture sites has been rendered insensitive by repeated venepuncture and anaesthesia is not required. If it is, placement of Emla cream (an emollient mixture including local anaesthetic) patches at proposed needle entry sites for 60 minutes before inserting the needle reduces the discomfort of the procedure. In general, there is little benefit to be obtained from injection of local anaesthetics because this itself involves insertion of a needle.

Procedure

- Swab generously with alcohol or iodine solution (providing the patient has no allergy to iodine or simply clean the arm with soap and water).

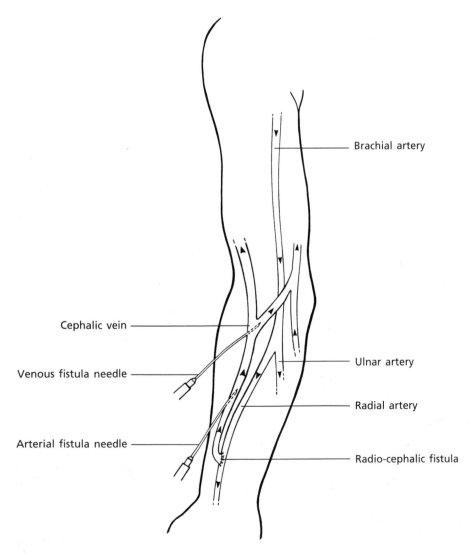

Figure 1.5 Positioning of needles for haemodialysis.

- The direction in which the access needle points is immaterial. Insert the needle over the fistula site or slightly to one side and advance it until a 'plop' is felt as the needle enters the vessel. Advance the needle until its hub is adjacent to the skin. Draw back gently on the syringe. If blood flows freely, empty the heparinized saline into the vein and clamp the tube. It is of no significance whether the 'arterial' access or the 'venous' access is established first. Ideally, flow from the 'arterial' access should be sufficient to push the plunger of the syringe back under its own force. The identical procedure is carried out for the 'venous' (return) needle, although in this case powerful flow sufficient to move the plunger of the syringe is not essential. The venous return needle should be proximal (cephalad) to the arterial needle (Figure 1.5). If satisfactory blood flow is not obtained on drawing back on the syringe, the vein may have been missed or cross-punctured. In either case, withdraw the fistula needle and press firmly on the exit site for 2–3 minutes before re-attempting cannulation. If blood clots appear in the access catheter or syringe (usually a consequence of too slow an attempt at needling), do the same and employ a new needle and catheter for a repeat attempt.
- Place the arterial and venous needles as far apart as possible to reduce the risk of recirculation of blood through the dialyser on more than one occasion.
- Connect the arterial end of the blood flow to the cannula.
- When blood has circulated through the artificial kidney (dialyser), insert the cannula into the venous female lock.
- Tape down the fistula needle using a winged Micropore method (Figure 1.6).

Removal of fistula needles
- Clamp the 'arterial' line and use the blood pump to return blood through the 'venous' line to the patient. When complete, clamp the venous line.

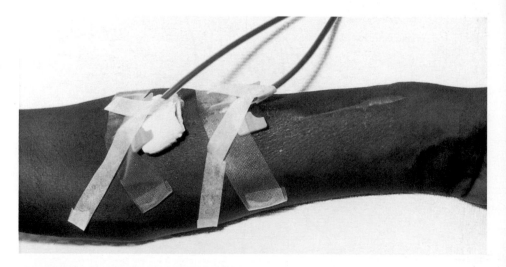

Figure 1.6 Cannulae in place and taped down.

- Remove needles, exert gentle pressure on the exit site for 1–5 minutes until bleeding ceases. Apply the gauze and tape down gently.

Persistent bleeding from fistula exit site

Firm pressure with a gloved finger applied to a gauze swab over the site will usually suffice. Avoid pressing too hard, which may promote clotting in the fistula. If this fails:

- Fill the cap of a universal container (diameter 2 cm approx.) fully with cotton wool.
- Place the cap (cotton wool down) over the site.
- Tape firmly in place (Figure 1.7) and apply a crêpe bandage, twisting the bandage each time it crosses the cap in order to apply pressure specifically over the bleeding site.

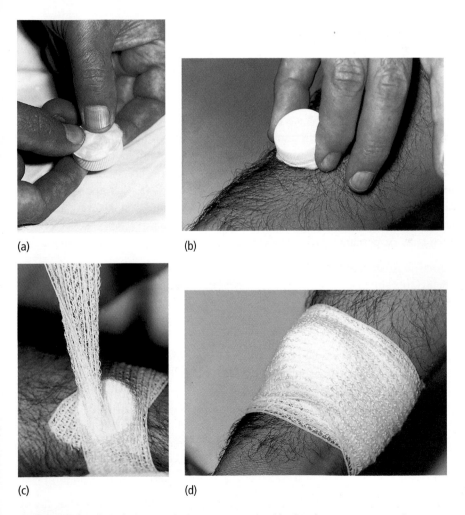

(a)

(b)

(c)

(d)

Figure 1.7 (a–d) Technique to deal with persistent bleeding from arteriovenous fistula. Note criss-cross arrangement of tape to exert maximum pressure on bleeding point.

chapter 2

VASCULAR ACCESS FOR HAEMODIALYSIS

This includes temporary access (central venous catheters and external arteriovenous shunts), long-term (tunnelled) central venous catheters and native arteriovenous fistulae and grafts.

TEMPORARY CENTRAL VENOUS ACCESS

Introduction

In this connection the term 'temporary' may mean vascular access destined to last from several hours to many weeks. Such access is required for haemodialysis and haemofiltration in which blood circulates through an artificial kidney (dialyser) or haemofilter. If the motive force for such blood circulation is the pumping action of the heart, arterial access will be required to remove blood from the patient and venous access to return it. If a mechanical pump is to be employed, arterial access is not required. Venous access is thus appropriate for haemodialysis and for pumped haemofiltration systems, and arterial access is needed for arteriovenous haemofiltration.

Three sites of percutaneous venous access are available:

- Internal jugular vein
- Subclavian vein
- Femoral vein.

Jugular access is preferable to subclavian for several reasons:

- Lower incidence of pneumothorax and haemothorax.
- Accidental puncture of carotid artery can be dealt with by direct pressure but subclavian artery puncture cannot.
- Subclavian venous catheters frequently cause venous stenosis (Figure 2.1), whereas for reasons that are unclear this is a much less frequent problem with jugular venous catheterization. Fashioning of an arteriovenous fistula on the side of a subclavian vein stenosis will often result in gross swelling of the arm owing to impaired venous return of blood from the arteriovenous fistula (Figure 2.2).

Jugular vein access does carry the disadvantage that infection, both local and systemic, is more likely than with subclavian access, but the disadvantages of the latter override this consideration.

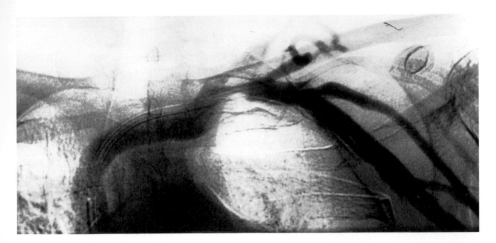

Figure 2.1 Venogram showing subclavian vein stenosis at the site of catheter entry into vein.

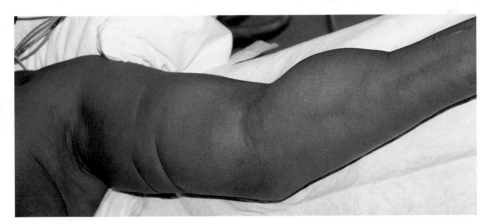

Figure 2.2 Gross swelling of the arm following formation of an arteriovenous fistula in a patient with ipsilateral subclavian vein stenosis.

It is preferable to access the right rather than the left internal jugular vein for the following reasons:

- The right internal jugular takes a straight course direct to the superior vena cava, whereas a catheter inserted into the left internal jugular vein has to pass through the innominate vein, therefore taking an angulated course.
- The apex of the pleura is lower on the right side.
- A left-sided jugular approach carries the risk of injury to the thoracic duct.

The femoral vein is suitable only for very short-term use, as there are considerable risks from infection and thrombosis, and a temporary catheter at this site also limits patient mobility. A femoral catheter may be useful if a single dialysis session with removal of the catheter is appropriate, as it may be in the case of a septic patient in whom bacterial colonization of a catheter inserted for longer term use is a risk.

Femoral venous access is also useful if internal jugular or subclavian vein catheterization fails or if the risk of bleeding is high. The femoral is the easiest appropriate vein to puncture and its location allows bleeding to be controlled readily by external compression.

The modern temporary dialysis catheter has a dual lumen construction that allows the use of a conventional blood circuit. The earlier generation of catheters were of single lumen design and are suitable only for a 'single needle' haemodialysis system. Single lumen catheters are cheaper and of smaller diameter. All types of catheter are manufactured to various lengths so that the procedure can be tailored to patient build. In general, a left-sided internal jugular or subclavian approach demands a longer catheter than a right-sided approach.

A recent improvement is a dual-lumen catheter designed specially for insertion into the internal jugular vein. This catheter has the hub end fashioned into a U-shape so that the catheter connectors are directed downwards, rather than upwards towards the patient's ear. The catheter is thus more comfortable for the patient and more stable (Figure 2.3).

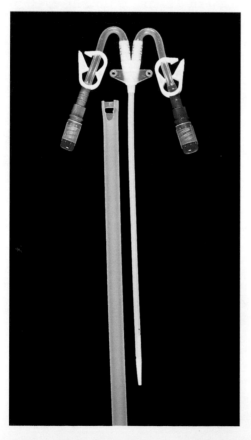

Figure 2.3 Jugular catheter with hub end fashioned into a U-shape for greater comfort and stability.

INSERTION OF INTERNAL JUGULAR VEIN CATHETERS

The method of choice employs ultrasound imaging of jugular vein and carotid artery such as the 'Site-rite' ultrasound scanner (Dymax Corp., Pittsburgh, USA). This technique is described first. Ultrasound equipment is not universally available and 'blind' jugular vein canulation, although less desirable, is also described.

Cannulation of the right internal jugular vein

Pre-procedure assessment

- Take a history of previous venous access. If the patient has a history of previous line insertion(s) or of difficulty in central venous access, ultrasound-guided line insertion is of particular value. If the necessary equipment is unavailable in the renal unit, ultrasound assessment or venography in the radiology department is advisable.
- Check haemoglobin, prothrombin time, platelet count, partial thromboplastin time with kaolin and bleeding time. Correct any abnormalities detected.
- Ensure that the patient is adequately hydrated prior to catheter insertion. Venous access is rendered much more difficult if veins are collapsed in a volume-depleted patient. Blood pressures should, if possible, be checked lying and standing immediately before cannula insertion. Postural hypotension, if present, is the signal to correct hypovolaemia before attempting the procedure.

Equipment

A sterile technique throughout the procedure is of paramount importance. Many catheter-associated infections are caused by organisms introduced at the time of insertion. Your trolley should contain the following items:

- Sterile towel with which to dry your hands.
- Sterile gown and gloves, and sterile drapes.
- Alcohol or iodine in a pot to clean skin.
- Several gauze swabs.
- Syringe containing 10 ml of 1–2 per cent lignocaine without adrenaline with one orange and one green needle. (The term 'orange' needle refers to the product by Microlance, 25 gauge A ⅝, 0.5 × 16 needle. The term 'green' needle refers to the Microlance 21 gauge 1½, 0.8 × 40 needle.)
- 5 ml syringe containing 5 ml of normal saline with an introducer needle.
- 20 ml syringes of normal saline.
- Guide-wire (check which is the 'soft end' and adjust it so that is ready for insertion through the introducer needle).
- Scalpel blade.
- Vessel dilator.
- Dual-lumen catheter. The 'red end' (arterial limb) ends a few centimetres proximal to the tip and the clip should be closed. The 'blue end' (venous

limb) ends at the tip of the catheter and the clip should be left open so that the guide-wire can pass through it. The lines come in two different lengths: usually the shorter 13.5 cm line is used in the first instance. The longer line is 19.5 cm long.

- Suture.
- Two 2 ml syringes each containing 1.5 ml of heparin 5000 units per ml. These are used to flush the arterial and venous limbs of the catheter.
- Empty 10 ml syringe with which to check blood flow rates.
- 10 ml syringe filled with normal saline.
- Micropore tape.
- Translucent dressing.
- Ultrasound scanner and probe, if employed.

Positioning the patient

The position of the patient is vital – if the patient is in an awkward position it may not be possible to find the vein. Explain the procedure precisely and then position the patient in a supine position with arms by the sides, lying straight on the bed, preferably with no pillows. Place the patient in a head-down posture, thus using gravity to distend the internal jugular vein, rendering initial puncture easier and reducing the risk of air embolism. You will need to stand behind the head of the patient, so remove the head of the bed. The head of the patient is turned away from the side of insertion, thus exposing the triangles of the neck. A small pillow may be used to extend the patient's neck slightly.

Anaesthetic

Lignocaine 1–2 per cent without adrenaline should be used.

Procedure

Prior to skin preparation, the jugular vein should be examined with the ultrasound probe to confirm position, size and patency. The carotid artery should also be indentified. The vein is readily compressed by exerting light pressure over the skin using the probe, whereas the artery is non-compressible. The jugular vein dimensions may be markedly increased by having the patient perform the Valsalva manoeuvre. This is best explained by asking the patient to hold his or her breath whilst pretending to strain at stool.

The ultrasound probe should normally be fitted with a 1.5 cm depth needle guide. Orientate the probe transversely to the neck with the needle guide pointing superiorly. With the scanner set to the 4 cm (actual size) view, keep the probe perpendicular to the skin and place it immediately superior to the clavicle. Maintain skin contact but do not apply pressure with the probe in case the vein collapses. Scan the length and breadth of the sterno-cleido-mastoid triangle, and observe where the vein is best seen at maximum diameter and/or at its greatest separation from the carotid artery.

Wash your hands meticulously with antiseptic solution and put on gown and gloves in the conventional sterile manner. With the patient in position, clean the skin with antiseptic solution, drape the sterile towels and dry the skin.

The basic principle is to puncture the vein with an introducer needle, advance a spring metal guide-wire, create a track with a vessel dilator and then insert the catheter over the wire.

Apply ultrasound gel to the end window of the probe and cover the probe with a sterile sheath, securing with elastic bands. Any wrinkles or bubbles over the acoustic window should be smoothed out with a gloved finger. Complete the acoustic coupling by wetting the patient's skin with copious amounts of sterile saline (sterile gel may be used if available). Hold the probe, cigar style, between the first two fingers of the non-dominant hand, with the needle guide to palm side, facing the operator. In this position the thumb will be found readily to fit into the half-moon cut-out of the needle guide (Figure 2.4). Initially, however, the thumb should be placed immediately above the needle-guide block for comfortable support during the preliminary phase.

Visualize the chosen entry point again and administer local anaesthetic directly below the 'V' of the needle guide. Using a no. 11 blade, make a nick in the skin at the same point. Place the tip of the needle in the incision, just through the skin and no more. Now bring the shaft of the needle up into the groove in the needle guide and trap it by placing the ball of the thumb firmly in the cut-out. When correctly done, the needle and syringe will be found to be self-retaining with this one-handed grip, leaving the other hand free to control the syringe. Ensure that the probe is perpendicular to the skin and watch the screen – not the neck! Centre the dotted target line over the vein, clear of the artery. Draw on the syringe plunger and, with constant aspiration, advance the

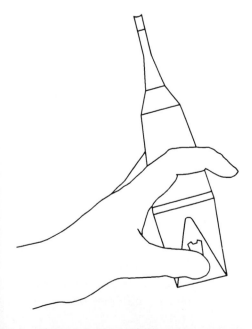

Figure 2.4 Ultrasound probe held in the non-dominant hand. Note position of thumb.

needle with a short stabbing motion. Bear in mind that the distance from the start position, just inside the skin, to the anterior aspect of the vein will be barely 1 cm; there is a tendency on first using the techinique to plunge too deeply too fast. With a conscious, co-operative patient, it may be helpful to request that the Valsalva manoeuvre be carried out by the patient, which increases the dimensions of the vein and the pressure within it, rendering puncture easier.

Should any difficulty be encountered in feeding the guide-wire at the 60 degree angle established by the needle guide, simply re-attach the syringe and drop the needle back to a more conventional angle whilst aspirating to confirm that the tip is still in the lumen.

As the needle is advanced, the anterior wall of the vein is seen to deform and invaginate, springing back as the needle penetrates the wall. Simultaneously, blood will be aspirated into the syringe. Note that steady, slow pressure as the needle is advanced may result in the anterior wall being compressed against the posterior wall before puncture takes place. In this situation, double-wall puncture may occur and the needle will have to be withdrawn into the lumen of the vein; this may be seen as an upward 'tenting' of the posterior wall.

Once the vein is punctured, the syringe/needle combination is supported by the dominant hand while the probe is laid down. The sub-dominant hand is then returned to the needle hub, the syringe removed and the guide-wire inserted.

Once the introducer needle is in the vein, keep the needle still in relation to the patient while carefully removing the syringe. Have the guide-wire ready and put the soft or 'J' end down through the needle. Avoid blood loss or air embolism using your thumb or finger on the end of the needle while carrying out this procedure. The guide-wire should be inserted smoothly and should encounter no resistance. If resistance is encountered, **do not force the wire**. If small alterations in the position of the needle do not solve the problem, remove the guide-wire, put the syringe back on the needle, check that the needle is still in the vein, adjust the position of the needle a little, check that it is still in the vein and then try the guide-wire again.

Assuming the guide-wire is in place, insert it 10–15 cm and then remove the introducer needle, leaving the guide-wire in position. Use the scalpel blade to make a 'stab' incision at the site of the guide-wire. Take care not to cut the wire by cutting away from it. The incision should be 3–4 mm wide and deep enough (5 mm) to penetrate subcutaneous tissues. Then take the dilator and insert it over the guide-wire, ensuring that the end of the guide-wire is not lost accidentally. Hold the end of the guide-wire with one hand, while the dilator is inserted with the other. A little pressure is required for the dilator to penetrate the subcutaneous tissues. Apply this by holding the dilator at a point close to the skin and exerting a small constant pressure.

If undue pressure is required, this may be as a result of kinking of the guide-wire. Check that this is not the case by moving the wire a few millimetres out and in within the dilator – it should move freely. If the wire becomes irreversibly kinked, there is no option but to remove it and insert a different one.

It will become obvious that the dilator is in the vein if, after a few centimetres of insertion, there is no resistance. If this is the case, remove the dilator, keeping the guide-wire in place, and ensuring that you retain a grip on the guide-wire and do not allow it to enter the patient's venous system. In a thin patient, there may be a little blood loss around the guide-wire which need not be a matter of concern. Take the dual-lumen catheter, the limbs of which are filled with normal saline, and insert it over the guide-wire using the blue (venous) limb. The catheter should pass over the guide-wire with no resistance and should not be forced. Once in the vein, blood may be seen in the catheter around the guide-wire. Continue the introduction of the catheter over the wire, again without releasing hold of the wire, until it is fully inserted, then remove the guide-wire and clip shut the blue limb. The catheter is designed so that flows are usually best when the blue limb is above the red limb (i.e. at the head end), so insert it this way round.

Using an empty syringe, check the flows from each limb. In so doing, you will remove the air from the limbs and avoid re-injecting this air. Then flush both limbs with normal saline and fill them with 1.5 ml of heparin (5000 units/ml). Put the caps on the ends of the catheter. Infiltrate local anaesthetic adjacent to the exit site of the catheter and suture the catheter into place. Clean the skin, cover the insertion site with a translucent air-occlusive dressing, move the patient up to a sitting position and clean up the trolley (taking responsibility for all 'sharps').

Postoperative care
A chest X-ray should be carried out immediately after jugular catheter insertion to check that the position of the catheter is appropriate. Except in an emergency, the catheter should not be used until this has been done. During subsequent use (usually by nursing staff), a strict aseptic technique must be employed, the exit site treated with antiseptic (preferably an iodine-containing one) and a new occlusive dressing applied after use. Purulent discharge from the exit site should be swabbed and sent for culture. Reddening of skin along the line of the catheter, suggesting infection, should prompt antibacterial therapy.

Blind jugular vein cannulation
The internal jugular vein lies within the carotid sheath lateral to the carotid artery and behind the lateral border of the sternocleidomastoid muscle. It is most superficial to the skin in the space between the sternal and clavicular heads of the sterno-cleido-mastoid muscle. Approaches to the vein can be 'high', at the midpoint of the sterno-cleido-mastoid muscle (Figure 2.5) or 'low', between the two heads of the sterno-cleido-mastoid muscle (Figure 2.6). A 'low' approach is described here.

Identify the two heads of the sterno-cleido-mastoid muscle, one arising from the sternum and the other from the clavicle. These two heads join to form the apex of a triangle. With the patient in the position described, the jugular vein

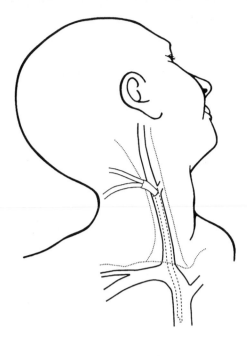

Figure 2.5 High approach to the internal jugular vein.

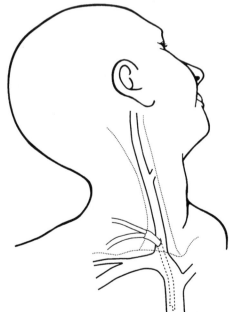

Figure 2.6 Low approach to the internal jugular vein.

will lie just below the apex. The carotid artery can usually be palpated easily, running medial to the vein. Infiltrate the skin at the apex of the triangle with local anaesthetic. With the fingers of your left hand (assuming you are right-handed), palpate the carotid artery. Infiltrate local anaesthetic using a green needle and, starting at the apex of the triangle just lateral to the carotid pulse, make a small stab incision with your scalpel. Aim the needle at 45 degrees to the skin towards the ipsilateral nipple. The jugular vein at this point is superficial and can always be found within the depth of a green needle. If the vein is not encountered, change the angle of approach. If the vein cannot be found with a green needle, it is no more likely to be found with the introducer needle. Assess whether venous or arterial blood is issuing. Thereafter, the technique is as described previously.

Complications

Inability to access the internal jugular vein
Small changes in the position of the patient can be very helpful. Check that the patient is lying in a symmetrical manner. Try removing the pillow, if present, and increase the head-down posture (if the patient is volume-depleted this can be very helpful, but the insertion should not be attempted under these circumstances). If these manoeuvres fail, do not persist until patient and operator become exasperated and demoralized. Either attempt to cannulate a different vein or, better still, request assistance (preferably from a more experienced or skilled operator).

Poor blood flow
Satisfy yourself that the catheter is in the vein, i.e. that there is at least some flow. If doubt remains, remove the catheter. If the patient is volume-depleted, give normal saline to render the patient euvolaemic. If the patient is volume-replete, try moving the catheter in or out a few millimetres, or rotating it a few degrees. If this fails, 'reverse' the catheter, i.e. re-insert the guide-wire, remove the catheter and re-insert it over the guide-wire with the red limb above the blue. If flow remains poor, consider changing the catheter for a longer one (using the guide-wire in a similar way). If flow remains poor, remove the catheter.

Inadvertent arterial puncture
Always consider actively when you enter a vessel whether it is a vein or an artery. The colour of blood obtained is an unreliable guide but the flow rate is extremely reliable. No venous flow is capable of filling a syringe unaided and no vein can pump blood on to your gown! If you are unsure about whether you are in an artery or vein, assume you are in an artery. Remove the needle and exert pressure for approximately 5 minutes over the puncture site. If the diagnosis of arterial puncture is missed and the catheter is inserted into the carotid artery, surgical removal and vessel repair may be indicated.

Pain
Pain arising from insufficient or misplaced local anaesthetic is easily rectified. Pain occurring as you insert the catheter is of more serious concern. Mild discomfort as the dilator is inserted is relatively common, but severe pain should alert you to the possibilities of pneumothorax and vessel rupture. If in doubt, stop the procedure.

Bleeding

External bleeding is relatively common and generally responds to local pressure. Using the minimum amount of extracorporeal anticoagulation may be of value. However, internal bleeding can be more sinister and may result in upper airways obstruction. This is an acute emergency that demands surgical intervention. Endotracheal intubation may be required.

Pneumothorax

The proximity of the pleura to both the internal jugular and subclavian veins means that there is a risk of causing a pneumothorax. Small pneumothoraces merely require observation, but a more sizeable one should be treated along conventional lines by chest drain insertion.

Haemothorax

Haemothorax can occur in isolation or associated with a pneumothorax. A large collection will require drainage and in severe cases a thoracotomy may be required.

Air embolism

Air embolism is a rare complication and is preventable by placing the patient in the correct head-down position. If it occurs, place the patient in a left lateral, head-down posture and institute basic resuscitation as required. Intensive care and even hyperbaric therapies may be required in severe cases.

Cardiac arrhythmias

If the guide-wire or catheter comes into contact with the endocardium, cardiac arrhythmias can occur. This is an indication that the catheter or wire has been advanced too far. They are generally transient, but more serious arrhythmias, such as ventricular tachycardia or fibrillation, may occur.

Cardiac tamponade

Cardiac tamponade can result if the myocardial wall is penetrated by either the guide-wire or by the catheter. It is a serious complication with a high mortality.

Fractured guide-wire

The guide-wire consists of a flexible central core around which is wound a second finer wire which acts as a spring. The two wires are only bonded together at the ends to allow movement between the central core and its outer wrapping when the whole assembly is flexed. This construction gives the guide-wire its spring-like property, while preserving strength and flexibility. However, it is possible to fracture either wire, resulting in the outer one unwinding and jamming in either the introducer needle, vessel dilator or catheter. When this occurs, the whole assembly should be removed without pulling on the wire.

Very rarely, both wires are fractured, resulting in a segment of wire detaching into the central venous circulation, or even entering the pulmonary artery.

Generally, the lost piece of wire can be retrieved using an interventional radio-logical technique. A thoracotomy is rarely required.

Cannulation of the left internal jugular vein
This is carried out exactly as for right internal jugular cannulation, except for the fact that the patient's head is turned to the right. The technique is more difficult and hazardous than right internal jugular insertion.

INSERTION OF SUBCLAVIAN VEIN CATHETERS

Introduction
Right-handed patients who require regular haemodialysis will prefer fashioning of an arteriovenous fistula in the left arm, leaving the dominant arm free during haemodialysis sessions. Since subclavian cannulation may result in subclavian vein stenosis with engorgement of the arm owing to poor venous drainage after fashioning of an arteriovenous fistula, the right subclavian route is the preferred one for right-handed patients who are likely to require regular haemodialysis.

Preoperative assessment, equipment, positioning of the patient and anaesthesia are as previously described under 'Insertion of internal jugular vein catheters'.

Procedure employing ultrasound technique
The subclavian vein lies anterior to the subclavian artery, arising in the axilla and entering the thorax by passing over the first rib behind the sternal end of the clavicle. The site of insertion should be at a point two-thirds of the way along the clavicle towards the lateral end and just below it.

The ultrasound technique is very similar to that described for jugular vein visualization but with one significant difference. In the foregoing instructions for the internal jugular vein, the importance of maintaining the probe perpendicular to the skin was stressed. This is because the best ultrasound images of vessels are obtained when the ultrasound beam strikes the vessel at right angles; since the internal jugular runs parallel to the skin, this is achieved by keeping the probe upright.

In the case of the subclavian vein, the vessel lies deeper as it is followed laterally. Therefore, the image may be improved by tilting the probe head fore and aft while keeping it in contact with the skin.

The probe should be fitted with a 2.5 cm needle guide. The operator stands to the side of the patient, ipsilateral to the vessel to be punctured. The probe is orientated with the needle guide facing laterally, towards the operator.

The area of the delto-pectoral groove, just inferior to the lateral third of the clavicle, is scanned and the subclavian vein and artery visualized. On screen, these will appear with the artery to the left and the vein to the right (on the patient's right side; vice-versa on the left side). The anatomical orientation is actually artery superior, vein inferior; moving the probe inferiorly–superiorly will give the operator the sense of how the image relates to the underlying structures.

The artery and vein are distinguished by applying pressure to the skin with the probe; the vein may be readily compressed, while the artery remains patent and pulsatile. The technique for puncturing the vein is thereafter as described previously. Note that the needle is passing through layers of fascia anterior to the vessel; these may sometimes be seen to indent as the needle passes through them, confirming the position of the needle point.

If the vein lies significantly deeper than 2.5 cm, then the point of intersection of the needle tip with the vein may lie outside the echo beam and the typical invagination of the vessel wall may not be seen. However, provided that the course of the vein has been demonstrated to continue medially without deviation, this need not impede venepuncture. With the target line centred over the vein, continue to advance the needle with constant aspiration until blood is obtained.

The remainder of the procedure is as described under 'Insertion of subclavian vein catheters'.

Blind cannulation of the right subclavian vein

Using an orange needle, infiltrate lignocaine subcutaneously and generously. After 2 minutes, use the green needle to infiltrate local anaesthetic more deeply. Insert the green needle along the same track as will be used later to insert the introducer needle. First, pass beneath the clavicle so that the needle is being inserted upwards, i.e. parallel to the midline. Once beneath the clavicle (i.e. after about 0.5 cm), rotate the needle and syringe and advance straight towards the suprasternal notch. Use a thumb on the notch to ensure that the needle is pointing in the correct direction; the needle should be just beneath the clavicle. As you advance, you should be attempting gently to withdraw the syringe at all stages, so that you will know if a vessel has been entered. Every 0.5 cm, cease advancing and inject about 0.5 ml of local anaesthetic. In a small slim person, the green needle may well enter the vein, in which case lignocaine must not be injected. If the vein is not encountered, the likely explanation is that the green needle is not long enough. Withdraw the green needle and take up the introducer needle together with a 10 ml syringe containing a few millilitres of saline. Following exactly the route that was taken with the green needle, insert the introducer needle, again drawing on the syringe as it advances. After a few centimetres, the vein should be encountered. Once it is, advance another 3–5 mm so that the needle is fully in the vein and then stop, checking first that the needle is still in the vein. The remainder of the procedure is as described under 'Cannulation of the right internal jugular vein'.

Postoperative care and complications and their management are as previously described under 'Insertion of internal jugular vein catheters'.

Cannulation of the left subclavian vein is as described for right subclavian vein cannulation except that the patient's head is rotated to the right.

INSERTION OF FEMORAL VEIN CATHETERS

Introduction

The femoral vein lies medial to the femoral artery which itself lies medial to the femoral nerve in the inguinal region. The technique is to aim medial to the femoral pulse, towards the umbilicus, puncturing the vein just below the inguinal ligament.

Preoperative assessment, equipment and anaesthesia are as set out under internal jugular and subclavian vein cannulation.

Positioning of the patient

The patient lies supine with arms at the sides, either flat or with one pillow, if necessary, under the head. Ultrasound-guided access may be employed as described for internal jugular and subclavian access.

Procedure

Prepare the skin with disinfectant and drape with sterile towels. Infiltrate the proposed puncture site with local anaesthetic and make a small stab incision with your scalpel. Puncture the vein with an introducer needle (with syringe attached) and ensure that venous rather than arterial blood is being aspirated. Advance the guide-wire through the needle so that at least 15 cm of wire has entered the vein. If any resistance is encountered, withdraw the wire a short distance and try again. Do not under any circumstances force the wire to advance. Once the wire is in place, remove the introducer needle leaving the wire *in situ*.

Next dilate a track for the catheter by passing a dilator along the wire using a gentle rotating action. Whenever either a dilator or a catheter are passed along a guide-wire, it is important to check that the wire does not become jammed as there is a risk of the wire breaking off into the circulation. If the wire does

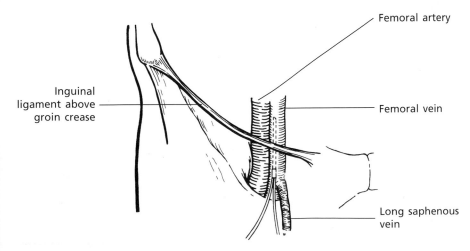

Figure 2.7 Haemodialysis catheter in right femoral vein.

become jammed, withdraw the wire and dilator/catheter together and repeat the procedure with a new wire via a fresh puncture.

Once satisfied with the catheter (Figure 2.7), flush the lumina with normal saline and 'lock' with 1.5 ml of heparin (5000 units/ml). Unless the catheter is to be removed at the end of the dialysis session, it is advisable to secure it with a skin suture. Clean the skin with alcohol or iodine, dry with gauze and cover the insertion site with a translucent air-occlusive dressing.

Post-procedure care and complications are as described previously.

REMOVAL OF JUGULAR AND SUBCLAVIAN CATHETERS

The patient should lie supine or with the head slightly down, if possible, to minimize the risk of entry of air. Full aseptic precautions are required, and a gown, gloves and mask should be worn. Swab the exit site and surrounding area of the catheter with a suitable antiseptic. Using sterile forceps and scissors, cut the sutures anchoring the catheter to the skin. Withdraw the catheter smoothly with immediate pressure over the puncture site after removal, employing gauze swabs. Apply an air-occlusive dressing to seal the site.

REMOVAL OF FEMORAL CATHETERS

Proceed as above except that the patient is positioned slightly head up.

EXCHANGE OF TEMPORARY ACCESS CATHETERS ('RAIL-ROADING')

This procedure is performed when a temporary access catheter becomes blocked or if the flows are too sluggish to enable satisfactory dialysis to be performed. A guide-wire is passed down the lumen of the existing catheter, the catheter is removed over the guide-wire and a new catheter is inserted into the vein over the existing guide-wire. The procedure avoids the need for relocalization of the vein or the need to use a different vein.

Infected catheters should, in general, not be rail-roaded. There is a significant risk that the new catheter will become colonized even if appropriate antibiotic cover is used. Rarely, however, venous access may be so difficult that the balance of risks makes rail-roading less of a risk than attempting to place a new catheter elewhere.

If there is a suspicion that there is thrombus or clot at the end of the existing catheter, then passing a guide-wire may cause fragmentation and embolization. This may be subclinical, or may cause significant symptoms or signs. The morbidity is highest when the thrombus or clot is infected. Rail-roading should not therefore be attempted in these circumstances.

Catheters in any of the major veins (internal jugular, subclavian or femoral) may be exchanged in this way.

A trolley should be set up containing the following sterile equipment:

- Sterile drapes
- Dressing pack
- Gauze swabs
- Iodine or other suitable skin cleaning material
- Guide-wire
- Replacement dialysis catheter
- Suture material
- Syringes
- Heparin, saline and lignocaine
- Dressing to cover the replacement line.

The patient should be positioned on a trolley or bed, with the appropriate area exposed. If the central venous catheter to be exchanged is in the neck, the patient should be positioned head down. If the catheter is in the femoral vein, the patient should be head up.

The existing dressing and sutures holding the catheter *in situ* are removed. The procedure should from this point onwards be performed with a strict aseptic technique. The hands are washed thoroughly and sterile cap, mask and gown should be worn.

The existing line and surrounding skin are cleaned with iodine-soaked gauze swabs. Sterile drapes are positioned around the site. Even with the best possible cleaning in this way, it is difficult to ensure that the existing catheter is rendered fully sterile. Therefore, after handling the catheter, gloves should be changed immediately.

The cap of the 'venous' limb of the existing catheter is removed. The guide-wire is passed down this limb, and the existing catheter is removed with the guide-wire remaining *in situ*. The existing catheter is discarded. The new catheter is passed over the guide-wire and into the vein, following which the guide-wire is removed. Both limbs of the new catheter are aspirated (to ensure flow is adequate) and then flushed through with saline. If the catheter is not to be used immediately, the lines should be 'locked' with heparin (1.5 ml, 5000 units/ml), and the caps placed on the ends of the catheter. The new catheter is stitched in position, using lignocaine for local anaesthesia, and the insertion site is covered with a suitable dressing.

Risks and complications

The risks associated with this procedure are relatively small. Air embolus should be avoided by appropriate positioning of the patient. Rupture or damage to the vein should be avoided by careful handling of the guide-wire and avoiding using any force to insert the wire or the new line. Bleeding from the exit site is usually only slight and can be treated with local pressure alone. A chest X-ray to check the position of the line and to exclude a pneumothorax is not required as a routine and should only be performed if the procedure does not go smoothly.

The major risk associated with the procedure is the introduction of infection. It is difficult for the inexperienced operator to ensure that the guide-wire and the new catheter are kept sterile, but the importance of this cannot be overemphasized.

TEMPORARY ARTERIOVENOUS ACCESS USING EXTERNAL DEVICES

PERCUTANEOUS FEMORAL ACCESS

Introduction
Access to both arterial and venous systems is required when performing haemofiltration using a spontaneous (non-pumped) blood circuit, such as continuous arteriovenous haemofiltration (CAVH), and continuous or intermittent arteriovenous haemodialysis (CAVHD). This may be achieved either using percutaneous femoral lines or an arteriovenous shunt, although in a critical care environment the former is often the first line of access.

Preprocedure investigations
Haemoglobin, prothrombin time, platelet count, partial thromboplastin time with kaolin and bleeding time should be checked, although, on occasion, the procedure will need to be carried out in the face of abnormalities. Ensure that the patient is not volume-depleted (see p. 11).

Equipment
Although conventional 8 FG dialysis catheters can be used, special CAVH/CAVHD catheters are available. These are non-tapered, do not have any side holes and are supplied with a tapered vessel dilator to allow percutaneous placement over a guide-wire. This design is said to offer superior blood flows when using a spontaneous circuit.

Positioning the patient
The patient lies supine with the legs slightly apart, and the hip externally rotated. Ultrasound screening, while helpful, is not mandatory.

Anaesthetic
Infiltration of local anaesthesia, such as 1 per cent plain lignocaine without adrenaline, is used.

Procedure (without ultrasound guidance)
Prepare the skin in the groin area with a topical antiseptic, such as aqueous povidone iodine solution. Drape with sterile towels, but ensure that the umbilicus is visible as this is used as an aiming point.

Start with the arterial side by palpating the femoral artery in the groin approximately 2 cm below the inguinal ligament. Anaesthetize the skin, and make a small stab incision. Puncture the artery with the introducer needle (plus attached syringe) by aiming at the femoral pulse along a line pointing towards the umbilicus. Ideally the needle should enter the artery where it passes below the inguinal ligament. This is where the artery passes through the femoral canal and can therefore be more readily compressed against bone to achieve haemostasis when the catheter is removed.

Once into the vessel, check that arterial blood can be aspirated and feed down a guide-wire. If there is doubt as to whether the introducer needle is in the artery, blood gas analysis will be helpful. Withdraw the needle, leaving the guide-wire *in situ*. Dilate the tract with a vessel dilator first, then introduce the catheter over the wire. A gentle twisting action is often required to help get the tip of the dilator/catheter through the vessel wall. Finally, test the catheter with a syringe, flush with saline and secure in place with a skin suture. If the catheter is not to be used immediately, 'lock' the lumen with 1.5 ml of heparin (5000 units/ml).

The technique of femoral vein puncture has already been described. There are no special instructions associated with the use of dedicated CAVH/CAVHD catheters.

With both catheters inserted, apply a sterile self-adhesive air-occlusive dressing.

Postoperative care
No postoperative X-ray is required and the catheters can be used immediately. The patient should be monitored for signs of complications.

Immediate complications

Bleeding
Bleeding can occur from both the arterial and venous sites, particularly if the patient is critically ill and has a concomitant coagulopathy. This can be managed by applying local pressure in the form of a pressure dressing and by using a minimum level of extracorporeal anticoagulation.

Arterial flow
An important complication is compromised arterial circulation to the leg, owing to disruption of atheromatous plaque, thrombosis, dissection or vascular steal. This is a serious complication that demands an early vascular surgical opinion.

ARTERIOVENOUS SHUNT

Introduction
An arteriovenous (A–V) shunt may be used when vascular access is required for immediate haemodialysis or haemofiltration. Now considered rather 'old-fashioned', it remains a valuable method of access. It allows blood flow through a dialysis or haemofiltration system without the need for a blood pump. The

alternative – percutaneous femoral arterial and venous puncture – has significant complications. However, shunt insertion requires some surgical skill, involves ligation of the artery that is used and may destroy potential sites for a future arteriovenous fistula. In recent years, the A–V shunt has largely been superseded by the use of percutaneous central venous catheters.

Preoperative assessment

A shunt may be inserted at the ankle (using the posterior tibial artery and long saphenous vein), the wrist (the radial artery and forearm cephalic vein) or, in extreme circumstances, the upper arm (the brachial artery and basilic vein). In desperation, any other suitable artery or vein may be cannulated. In all cases, the chosen artery must be easily palpable and the vein shown to be patent. Where possible, the other arteries providing distal blood supply should also be palpable, e.g. in the case of a radial artery shunt the ulnar artery should be palpable. In older patients who are hypotensive, flow through distal arteries (the posterior tibial and radial arteries) may not be adequate.

Equipment

A silastic shunt catheter with a Teflon tip is shown in Figure 2.8.

Position

Shunt insertion may be performed at the bedside, in a treatment room or in an operating theatre. The main prerequisite is good lighting. Having chosen the site for insertion, the skin is cleaned and draped in the standard way.

Anaesthesia

Direct infiltration of local anaesthetic – 1.0 per cent plain lignocaine – is usually adequate. Regional and general anaesthesia are rarely required.

Procedure

There are two aspects to the procedure: identification of the vessels, and cannulation with the shunt. Cannulation is performed in the same way regardless of

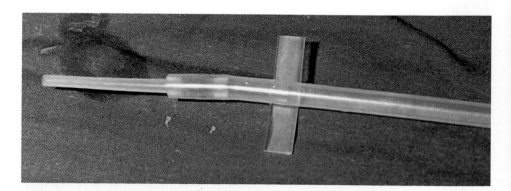

Figure 2.8 Silastic shunt catheter with Teflon tip.

which vessels are used. This will therefore be described 'in isolation' followed by a brief description of the exposure of the vessels at each of the three sites.

Vessel cannulation

The shunt is assembled and primed with normal saline. The vessel to be cannulated is exposed over a length of 2 cm and ligated distally with a 3/0 silk tie – the ends are left long. A second tie is positioned, but not tied, around the vessel proximally. The vessel is held between non-toothed dissecting forceps and a 2 mm opening made with a no. 11 blade. A Watson–Cheyne dissector is passed proximally up the vessel. The shunt tip is gently inserted into the vessel, initially at an angle of 90 degrees to the vessel, and advanced proximally. The proximal tie is ligated around the vessel containing the shunt tip. The distal tie is ligated around the shunt itself to hold it in place, and finally the proximal and distal ties are ligated together for further security. Free flow of blood into the vein or out of the artery is confirmed. The distal end of the shunt is brought out through a small stab incision. When both artery and vein have been cannulated, the two shunt limbs are connected and free flow confirmed (Figure 2.9).

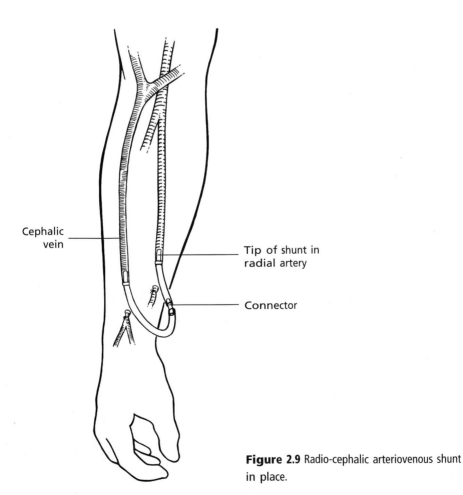

Cephalic vein

Tip of shunt in radial artery

Connector

Figure 2.9 Radio-cephalic arteriovenous shunt in place.

Vessel exposure

- The ankle. The transverse incision is made on the medial side of the leg 4 cm proximal to the medial malleolus and parallel to, but 1 cm posterior to, the anterior border of the tibia. The artery lies below the deep fascia in the neurovascular bundle between flexor digitorum longus anteriorly and flexor hallucis longus posteriorly. The vein lies in the fat below the anterior edge of the incision.
- The wrist. The incision is longitudinal, half way between the radial pulse and the cephalic vein. The artery is below the deep fascia and the vein is in the superficial fat.
- The upper arm. The longitudinal incision is directly over the brachial artery where it can be palpated medial to biceps, 4–5 cm proximal to the elbow. The artery lies below the deep fascia and care must be taken to avoid damage to the median nerve. There are usually two or three venae comitantes lying close to the artery which join into a single larger vein more proximally.

In all cases the wound is closed with interrupted nylon skin sutures.

Postoperative care

The shunt may be used immediately. Postoperatively, and after each use, the exit sites are cleaned with alcohol or an iodine solution, dried and covered with sterile gauze.

Complications

Local, and sometimes systemic, infection requires antibiotic treatment. Clotting, which may be predisposed to by hypotension, kinking of the shunt or infection, is the main complication. Declotting catheters – fine catheters that can be inserted through the shunt to the vessel – are available; these are used to extract thrombus. Gentle manipulation with a saline-filled syringe may be effective, although care must be taken to avoid excess pressure leading to embolization of fragments of thrombus.

LONG-TERM (TUNNELLED) CENTRAL VENOUS CATHETERS

Introduction

Long-term central venous access may be provided by a number of commercially available catheters (Figure 2.10).

These are dual-lumen catheters, made of silastic, and are available in a variety of lengths – 40 cm is the standard length for insertion into the right internal jugular vein, but both shorter and longer catheters are available. The catheter is placed in a subcutaneous tunnel and has a Dacron cuff attached designed to stimulate fibrous ingrowth from the surrounding tissues that both anchors the catheter in position and limits the spread of infection from the exit site to the point of entry into the vein.

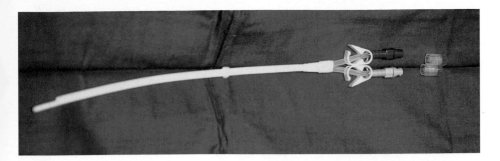

Figure 2.10 Catheter for longer term central venous access.

It is possible to use the internal jugular or subclavian veins. The jugular approach is preferred in view of the risk of subclavian vein stenosis, and the right jugular is preferred to the left because its course is shorter and for the reasons given on p. 9.

Tunnelled jugular catheters emerge just below the clavicle. Subclavian venous catheters have no bend and can be tunnelled at a slight angle to emerge between the clavicle and the nipple. The tunnel should be 10–12 cm long, depending on the patient and the catheter employed. If it is too short, it will not be a sufficient barrier to infection; if it is too long, it becomes more difficult to insert.

Tunnelled central venous catheters may provide satisfactory access for periods in excess of 1–2 years in patients whose vessels are inadequate to allow fashioning of an arteriovenous fistula. They are useful also when access is required for 2–3 months while waiting for permanent access to 'mature'.

Pre-procedure assessment

In a patient in whom no previous central venous catheter has been inserted, no specific preoperative investigation of the venous system is required. If previous catheters (short term or long term) have been used, there is a risk that the central veins may be stenosed or thrombosed. Ultrasonography or venography may be required to demonstrate patency of the vein intended as the site of insertion.

Haemoglobin, platelet count, prothrombin time and partial thromboplastin time with kaolin should be checked. Care should be taken to ensure that the patient is not volume-depleted prior to the procedure.

Equipment

A trolley laid up for the procedure is shown in Figure 2.11.

Positioning the patient

The catheter should be inserted in an operating theatre with full sterile precautions. The preferred site of insertion is the right internal jugular vein; the left internal jugular vein is the second-choice site, as there is more likelihood that

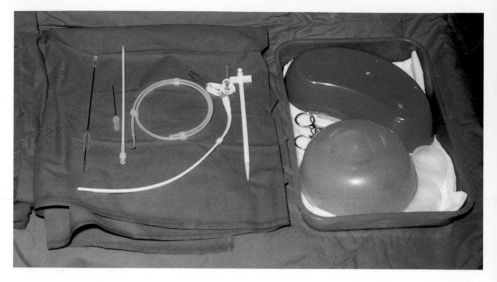

Figure 2.11 Trolley laid up for 'Permcath' insertion.

the catheter will be incorrectly positioned and there appear to be more complications using the left-sided approach. The neck is extended, if necessary, using a head ring and/or a sandbag placed between the patient's shoulder blades, and the head is rotated 45 degrees to the contralateral side.

CATHETER INSERTION UNDER GENERAL ANAESTHESIA

While catheter insertion may be performed using local anaesthesia, this is not always satisfactory or feasible. Endotracheal intubation or a laryngeal mask are equally acceptable; it is difficult to perform the operation if a facemask is used. The operating table should be tilted so that the patient is lying moderately head-down, to minimize the risk of air embolism during the procedure.

Procedure

The general principle of the operation is to position the catheter such that the tip is lying in the right atrium. The easiest and most direct route to the right atrium is via the right internal jugular vein and that procedure will be described in detail. Alternative entry sites are the right external jugular vein, and the internal and external jugular veins on the left side; the surgical procedure is modified accordingly, if necessary. The only significant anatomical difference affecting left-sided insertion is the thoracic duct, which enters the left internal jugular vein close to (usually inferior to) the site of exposure of the vein. It must be avoided, as a lymphatic fistula is a troublesome complication.

After antiseptic skin preparation, extending from the chin and mandible down to below the nipples, the operative area is draped in standard fashion, using a head towel. A transverse skin crease incision is made approximately 3 cm above the medial 3 cm of the clavicle, and parallel to the clavicle. Platysma is divided in the line of the incision, exposing the sternomastoid muscle. In thin patients it may be possible to separate the two heads of the muscle but more typically the muscle is cut transversely. The internal jugular vein is found lying below a layer of fascia. If obscured by muscle, this is retracted cranially. The vein can then be mobilized by sharp and blunt dissection, taking care not to damage small tributaries. Before making the subcutaneous tunnel, it is important to place the catheter on the patient's chest to estimate the correct length of catheter to be inserted into the vein, thus allowing an accurate estimation of the position of the exit site. A small stab incision is made at the exit site and the catheter passed through a subcutaneous tunnel from the exit site to the operative site. Both lumina are flushed with normal saline and clamped to ensure the catheter is free of air. It is also important to check that any small fat particles that may have entered the catheter from the subcutaneous tunnel are flushed out.

Two vascular clamps angled at 45 degrees are applied to the vein, their tips meeting to isolate an adequate length of vein. Using a no. 11 scalpel blade, a venotomy is made and enlarged to approximately 3 mm in diameter. A purse-string suture, using 5/0 Prolene, is placed around the venotomy. The catheter tip is inserted into the vein, the proximal (i.e. nearest the thorax) vascular clamp is removed and the catheter fed into the vein. Tension on the purse-string suture will usually control bleeding while free flow (in and out) of both lumina is checked using a syringe of normal saline. The position of the catheter should be checked using X-ray screening (fluoroscopy). The tip of the catheter should lie in the right atrium. The second vascular clamp is removed and the suture tied.

The sterno-mastoid and platysma muscles are sutured in two layers with chromic catgut, and the skin with subcuticular Dexon. The external part of the catheter is secured with a suture – but not at the exit site, to minimize the risk of exit-site infection – and both incision site and exit site are covered with sterile dressings.

Postoperative care

Following insertion, both lumina are filled with 1.5 ml of heparin (5000 units/ml). Priming volumes of catheters vary but are typically approximately 1.5 ml for each lumen. The catheter is filled with heparin following each dialysis.

It is standard practice to confirm the position of the catheter on a chest X-ray before first use.

Surgically inserted central venous catheters may be used immediately following insertion. Blood flow rates of at least 250–300 ml/minute should be possible, with a venous pressure normally less than 100 mmHg.

Complications

Significant surgical complications of catheter insertion are fortunately rare. Bleeding around the exit site may occur. This is normally caused by vessels in the subcutaneous tunnel, which are inaccessible, and is treated by local pressure. The two most significant complications are infection and blockage. Exit-site infections are minimized by careful skin care and immobilization of the catheter by a dressing to minimize movement at the exit site. Systemic sepsis associated with the catheter is a significant problem as eradication of sepsis without removal of the catheter may be impossible. One-way obstruction of the catheter (flow into the patient is possible but blood withdrawal is not) may occur if the tip of the catheter is lying tightly against the wall of the vein or if small thrombi form around the catheter tip. Gentle flushing with saline, changing the patient's position or even a large cough may resolve the problem. Urokinase, 25 000 units in 1.5 ml of normal saline, may be left in the catheter for 4–12 hours if simpler methods are unsuccessful. If no other solution is possible, the dialysis lines may be reversed, although this results in a significant increase in recirculation and reduction in dialysis efficiency.

CATHETER INSERTION UNDER LOCAL ANAESTHESIA

Pre-procedure assessment
This is as set out for surgical placement.

Equipment
This is shown in Figure 2.11.

Positioning the patient
The patient lies supine, and for internal jugular or subclavian vein cannulation is placed head-down. Ultrasound and X-ray screening are not mandatory but should be used if at all possible. The latter enables the catheter tip to be accurately positioned at the time of insertion, particularly as a tunnelled silicone rubber catheter cannot easily be manipulated after implantation.

Anaesthetic
This procedure is performed under infiltrated local anaesthesia, although in some cases intravenous sedation will be necessary. Use 1 per cent lignocaine without adrenaline or its equivalent.

Procedure
The basic technique is to introduce a guide-wire into the vein via a needle, dilate a track and insert a peel-away sheath. This enables the soft silicone rubber catheter to be fed into the vein, following which the sheath is peeled away leaving the catheter in place. The catheter is tunnelled subcutaneously before insertion into the vein.

The initial stages of this procedure, up to the introduction of the guide-wire, are identical to those described on pp. 19–20. It is usual to employ the 'low' approach to the internal jugular vein for this procedure. Once the guide-wire is in place, the skin incision is extended with a scalpel to approximately 2 cm in length, taking great care not to damage the wire. The next step is to fashion a subcutaneous tunnel. The catheter has a fixed hub assembly, which dictates that the catheter is tunnelled from the outside before feeding into the vein. The aim is to fashion an exit site lateral to the vein such that the Dacron felt cuff lies within the skin tunnel, approximately 2 cm from the surface. A good exit-site location is at the anterior chest wall in the infraclavicular fossa. In women, avoid tunnelling into breast tissue as this can create discomfort, and avoid the mid-clavicular line to prevent a bra strap rubbing on the exit site. It is helpful to use the catheter as a template for exit-site location, assuming that the tip will lie in the vicinity of the sternal angle. However, avoid excessive handling of the catheter to reduce the risk of bacterial contamination. Having chosen an exit-site location, infiltrate the skin with local anaesthetic and make a 5–8 mm stab incision. Draw the catheter through the exit site and through the first incision using a good-quality metal tunnelling tool.

Now insert a peel-away sheath plus dilator assembly into the vein using the guide-wire. This is quite a large device. Some makes have an oval cross-section to accommodate the catheter. If the sheath does not enter the vein easily, do not force it; instead, use smaller vessel dilators first (e.g. 8 FG) to dilate the track gradually. With the sheath in the vein, withdraw the vessel dilator and guide-wire, and occlude the end of the sheath with a gloved finger. Flush the catheter lumina with sterile saline and feed the catheter down the sheath, using X-ray screening to check that it is passing towards the right atrium. Peel the sheath apart, leaving the catheter in place and check the position using X-ray screening; the tip should lie in the superior vena cava, just above its junction with the right atrium (Figure 2.12). Now is the time to fine tune the catheter position and ensure

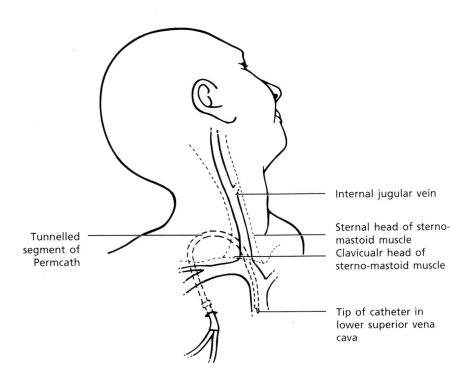

Internal jugular vein

Sternal head of sterno-mastoid muscle

Clavicualr head of sterno-mastoid muscle

Tunnelled segment of Permcath

Tip of catheter in lower superior vena cava

Figure 2.12 Tunnelled internal jugular Permacath – low approach.

there are no kinks in the tunnelled section. It is often necessary to perform some gentle blunt dissection to locate the cuff, using a small pair of artery forceps.

Before closing the skin incision, test each lumen with a 20 ml syringe. The syringe should readily fill in under 10 seconds (20 ml in 6 seconds represents a blood flow rate of 200 ml per minute). Flush both lumina with normal saline and 'lock' with 1.5 ml of heparin (5000 units/ml). Close the skin incision with one or two interrupted sutures and apply self-adhesive dressings to the wound and exit site.

If the left jugular or subclavian approach (Figure 2.13) is to be employed, the technique is modified as set out on pp. 19–20.

Until fibrosis has occurred into the Dacron felt cuff, there is a risk of displacing the catheter if external traction is accidentally applied. Particularly during the first 2–4 weeks, the catheter must be handled with extreme care. To reduce this risk it is possible to insert an additional securing suture around the catheter hub, and some makes have specific suture points for this purpose.

Postoperative care

Take a plain, erect, chest X-ray to check for pneumothorax or haemothorax, and to confirm the final catheter position prior to use. Monitor the patient for signs of complications and administer analgesia as required.

Remove any non-absorbable skin sutures on the 10th postoperative day.

Immediate complications

These include all of those described as associated with percutaneous temporary central venous access. The only additional immediate complication is bleeding

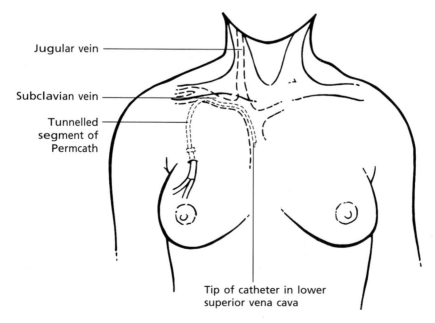

Jugular vein

Subclavian vein

Tunnelled segment of Permcath

Tip of catheter in lower superior vena cava

Figure 2.13 Tunnelled subclavian 'Permcath'. Note tip of catheter lies in superior vena cava just above junction with right atrium.

from the subcutaneous tunnel, which usually responds to the application of local pressure and rarely needs surgical intervention.

CHANGING TUNNELLED CENTRAL VENOUS CATHETERS

It is usually possible to change the catheter over a guide-wire without the need to expose the site of the venotomy. The catheter *in situ* is removed through an incision over the Dacron cuff, a guide-wire having been inserted before the catheter is removed. There is a 'pseudo-sheath' formed around the catheter and a new catheter, suitably positioned in a subcutaneous tunnel, will usually pass along the pseudo-sheath over the guide-wire.

REMOVAL OF TUNNELLED CENTRAL VENOUS CATHETERS

Introduction
The removal of both percutaneously and surgically implanted central venous catheters can be performed at the bedside on an outpatient basis.

Preparatory investigations
No specific preparatory investigations are required.

Positioning the patient
The patient lies supine and, in the case of internal jugular or subclavian catheters, in a slight head-down tilt to reduce the risk of air embolism.

Anaesthetic
Infiltration of local anaesthestic is used, such as 1 per cent plain lignocaine or an equivalent. The patient will very rarely need intravenous sedation.

Procedure
Palpate the catheter along its subcutaneous tunnel and identify the exact position of the Dacron felt cuff. Using an aseptic technique, infiltrate local anaesthetic into the skin over the cuff and into the tissues immediately around it, taking great care not to inject into or damage the catheter. Make a 1 cm skin incision over the cuff using a small scalpel, again taking care not to cut the catheter for the following reasons:

- If the wall is perforated through the lumen there is the risk of either blood escaping or air embolism.
- Once cut, silicone rubber tears easily and this may result in the catheter shearing off completely. This could lead to loss of the distal end into the central venous system.

Once the cuff is exposed, use blunt dissection with a pair of small artery forceps to free the cuff completely from its surrounding tissues. The end of the catheter distal to the cuff should now pull out readily and the remaining track down to the vein can be occluded by applying external pressure. Haemostasis should be achieved in about 5 minutes.

Finally, divide the catheter proximal to the cuff and simply pull the tunnelled section out. Close the skin incision with one or two interrupted sutures and apply self-adhesive dressings to seal the site and prevent the entry of air. The exit site does not require any sutures.

Postoperative care
Monitor for signs of complications, especially bleeding, and administer analgesia as required.

Remove any non-absorbable skin sutures on the 10th postoperative day.

Immediate complications

Bleeding
Treat by applying local pressure, and move the patient to a sitting position to reduce central venous pressure. Surgical intervention is very rarely needed.

Air embolism
Place the patient in a left lateral, head-down posture and institute basic resuscitation as required. Intensive care and even hyperbaric oxygen treatment may be required in more extreme cases.

Lost section of catheter
Where a section of catheter is lost in the skin tunnel, it is possible to extend the skin incision and retrieve it. If a piece of catheter is lost into the central venous circulation it can usually be retrieved by using an interventional radiological technique. Very occasionally, thoracic surgery may be required.

LONG-TERM VASCULAR ACCESS

NATIVE ARTERIOVENOUS FISTULA

Introduction
The native (i.e. using the patient's own vessels) arteriovenous fistula (AVF) is the standard form of vascular access for haemodialysis and is the first-choice procedure. The temptation to employ an arteriovenous prosthetic graft, simply because the procedure is considered simpler surgically, should be resisted. Where possible it should be fashioned at least 3 months prior to the need for haemodialysis to give time for the vein to 'mature'. If immediate dialysis is required, an alternative form of access must be used in the interim period. Whenever possible, the fistula should be fashioned in the non-dominant arm.

Preoperative assessment

It is essential to confirm that the artery to be used is easily palpable and that the vein is patent. The most successful fistulae develop when the vein is of good diameter, has few branches and runs up the arm in a relatively straight fashion. Clinical examination will usually allow the appropriate site for a fistula to be chosen. At times, preoperative ultrasonography or venography will be required. The classical AVF is created at the wrist using the radial artery and forearm cephalic vein. Frequently, however, the radial artery is inadequate as increasing numbers of older patients and those with diabetes enter haemodialysis programmes. The most common reason for an inadequate vein is prior use – often for an intravenous infusion – leading to thrombosis. If suitable vessels are absent from both forearms, it is necessary to consider fashioning an antecubital ('brachial') fistula.

There are usually two veins in the antecubital fossa – the median basilic and the more lateral upper arm cephalic vein. Only the cephalic vein makes a suitable fistula, as the median basilic vein passes deep into the arm just proximal to the antecubital fossa, and is inaccessible.

The patient must not be hypovolaemic. Physical examination, including blood pressure measurements taken when the patient is lying down and standing, will indicate the need for preoperative intravenous fluid.

The increasing use of short-term subclavian catheters has resulted in an increasing incidence of asymptomatic subclavian venous stenosis or thrombosis. The increased venous return that follows AVF formation may then cause severe oedema of the ipsilateral arm (Figures 2.1 and 2.2). If a patient has had multiple or prolonged subclavian cannulation on the side of the proposed fistula, assessment of the subclavian vein by ultrasound or venography is indicated preoperatively.

Positioning the patient

The procedure is performed in the operating theatre with full aseptic precautions. The arm is positioned on a small arm table, the skin cleaned and drapes applied.

Anaesthesia

Anaesthesia may be local, regional or general, depending upon the general condition of the patient and the experience of the anaesthetist. Some regional techniques fail to block the lateral cutaneous nerve of the forearm, which supplies the skin close to the site of a forearm fistula.

Procedure

Forearm fistula

The incision is longitudinal, between the radial artery and the forearm cephalic vein, immediately proximal to the radial styloid. Artery and vein must be mobilized for 4–5 cm such that they can lie side-to-side without tension. The

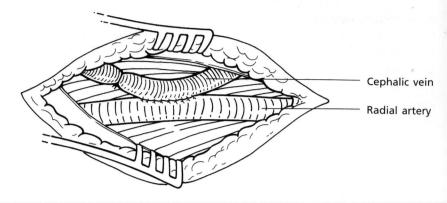

Figure 2.14 Side-to-side radio-cephalic arteriovenous fistula.

vessels are clamped proximally and distally, and opened on their anterior surfaces for approximately 2 cm. The anastomosis is performed using 6/0 Prolene. On completion of the anastomosis, but before ligation of the suture, a Watson–Cheyne dilator is passed distally and proximally up both artery and vein, whilst removing the vascular clamps, in order to dilate the vessels. The Prolene is then tied. A thrill should be palpable over the anastomosis and the proximal vein. A palpable pulse (but no thrill) over the vein suggests good arterial inflow but no venous run-off, whereas no pulse or thrill implies no arterial inflow. It is essential to ensure that the artery and vein are not kinked or tethered following the anastomosis and that there is no undue tension. If necessary, the vein may be ligated distally (Figure 2.14). Alternatively, an end-to-side fistula may be fashioned in the first place (Figure 2.15) Once satisfactory flow has been established, the wound is closed with interrupted nylon skin sutures.

Antecubital fistula

The preferred procedure is an end-to-side anastomosis between the upper arm cephalic vein and the brachial artery. A side-to-side anastomosis is technically

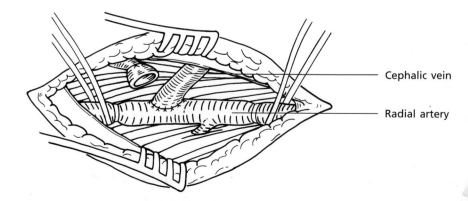

Figure 2.15 End-to-side radio-cephalic fistula.

more difficult and is likely to cause a swollen forearm as a consequence of retro-grade venous flow if the distal limb of the vein is left unligated. A transverse incision is made across the antecubital fossa. The vein is mobilized both proxi-mally and distally. It is important to ensure adequate mobilization to allow the vein to reach the brachial artery without tension or kinking. The vein is divided distally, the distal end ligated, and the proximal end controlled with a small 'bulldog' clamp. The brachial artery is mobilized over approximately 2–3 cm – this may involve partial division of the bicepital aponeurosis. The artery is clamped proximally and distally and a 1.0–1.5 cm arteriotomy made. The vein is spatulated up its medial surface and the end-to-side anastomosis performed with 6/0 Prolene (Figure 2.16). As before, the vessels are dilated using a Watson–Cheyne dilator prior to ligation of the suture. The flow is checked and, if satisfactory, the skin is closed with nylon sutures.

Postoperative care
The arm is wrapped in a warm towel for the immediate postoperative period. If necessary, flow may be encouraged by 500–1000 ml of normal saline given intravenously. It is essential that blood is not taken from the fistula arm and that no blood pressure cuff is applied to that arm. The fistula should be palpated or inspected with a stethoscope regularly in the first 12–24 hours. If flow stops abruptly, the patient should be taken back to the operating theatre immediately and the fistula re-explored. A forearm fistula can usually be used 6–8 weeks postoperatively, whereas a good brachial fistula may be ready within 4 weeks.

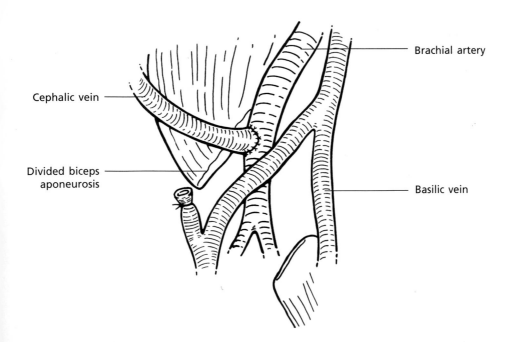

Figure 2.16 Right antecubital fistula.

Complications

Immediate postoperative complications are:

- Clotting – see above
- Bleeding – re-operation is usually required.

A detailed description of the long-term complications and their management is outside the scope of this chapter. The most commonly encountered problems are:

- Failure of the fistula to develop. This may result from inadequate arterial inflow or poor venous run-off.
- Aneurysm formation.
- Distal venous hypertension. This is more common following a side-to-side anastomosis at the wrist. Excessive flow into the distal vein may produce swelling, redness and skin changes over the thumb and/or first finger. This can be avoided in most cases by ligation of the distal vein at the initial procedure.
- Distal ischaemia. This usually takes the form of a 'steal' syndrome, is more common following an antecubital fossa fistula, and may require ligation of the fistula if severe. The severity of the vascular steal – and consequent pain – is usually greatest during haemodialysis treatment sessions.
- Swelling of the entire arm. As described above, this implies stenosis or thrombosis of the subclavian vein. If this cannot be corrected, ligation of the fistula may be required, following which the oedema usually settles rapidly.

ARTERIOVENOUS GRAFTS

Introduction

The first choice procedure for vascular access is the forearm arteriovenous fistula. The antecubital fossa fistula is a reasonable second-choice procedure. However, if all fistula sites have been used unsuccessfully or are unsuitable, a fistula may be created using some form of vascular graft. A number of 'biological' materials have been used (human umbilical vein, long saphenous vein, bovine carotid artery and bovine mesenteric veins) but most units now use a synthetic graft manufactured from expanded polytetrafluoroethylene (PTFE). A number of manufacturers produce satisfactory grafts in a variety of configurations: diameter 4–8 mm, length 15–80 cm, externally supported in their curved segment (to avoid kinking) and with a variety of wall types, each claiming to allow easier needle insertion and less post-dialysis bleeding.

Preoperative assessment

The advantage of a PTFE graft is that, while it is positioned subcutaneously (to allow needle insertion), the arterial and venous anastomoses may be to deeper vessels that are unsuitable or inappropriate for native arteriovenous fistula (AVF) creation. Clinical examination should confirm that an adequate arterial pulse is

Table 2.1 Typical PTFE graft sites

Arterial inflow	Venous run-off	Configuration	Site
Radial artery	Basilic cubital vein	Straight	Forearm
Brachial artery	Basilic cubital vein	Looped	Forearm
	Cephalic vein (in delto-pectoral groove)	Straight	Upper arm
	Axillary vein	Straight	Upper arm
	Subclavian vein	Straight	Upper arm
Axillary artery	Axillary vein	Looped	Upper arm
Superficial femoral artery	Femoral vein (superficial or common)	Looped/straight	Thigh
	Long saphenous vein	Looped/straight	Thigh

palpable at the proposed site of the anastomosis and that the distal arterial pulses are palpable. This is particularly important in patients at risk of peripheral vascular disease, e.g. diabetic and older patients, as the graft may produce a 'steal' syndrome leading to distal ischaemia in the presence of severe arterial disease. Duplex scanning, arteriography and/or venography may be required to establish vascular patency and to identify the preferred site for the anastomoses.

Equipment
A variety of PTFE grafts is shown in Figure 2.17.

Positioning the patient and the graft
There is no consensus as to the most appropriate site and configuration of a vascular graft. It may be positioned in the forearm, upper arm or thigh, and may run as a straight graft, e.g. from the radial artery at the wrist to a vein in the antecubital fossa, or as a curve, e.g. from the superficial femoral artery to the femoral vein, curving subcutaneously across the front of the thigh (Table 2.1). Examples of forearm 'loop' and brachio-axillary straight PTFE grafts are

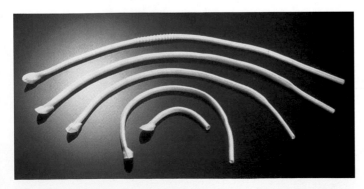

Figure 2.17 A variety of expanded polytetrafluoroethylene grafts.

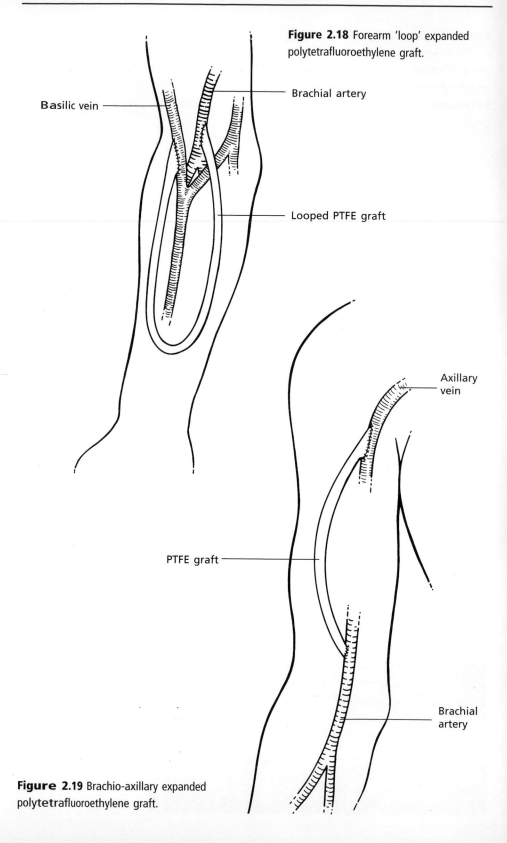

Figure 2.18 Forearm 'loop' expanded polytetrafluoroethylene graft.

Basilic vein

Brachial artery

Looped PTFE graft

Axillary vein

PTFE graft

Brachial artery

Figure 2.19 Brachio-axillary expanded polytetrafluoroethylene graft.

shown in Figures 2.18 and 2.19, respectively. In more extreme situations, a graft has been positioned across the upper chest from the axillary or subclavian artery to the contralateral subclavian or internal jugular vein. All procedures have in common the need: (a) for adequate arterial inflow and venous run-off; (b) to position the graft subcutaneously, close enough to the skin to allow easy needle insertion but deep enough to prevent skin necrosis over the graft; and (c) to ensure the graft does not cross a joint. All procedures are performed in the operating theatre under fully sterile conditions.

Anaesthesia
General anaesthesia is preferred as the procedures take longer to perform than simple arteriovenous fistula formation and usually involve more extensive dissection. However, good regional anaesthesia may be satisfactory for many arm – especially forearm – grafts.

Procedure
Because of the variety of sites and configurations, it is not possible to describe in detail every surgical procedure. However, the following general principles apply to all commonly used sites.

Both artery and vein are exposed and mobilized over an adequate length. The graft – usually 6 mm in diameter – is positioned in a subcutaneous tunnel, due care being taken to ensure that this is neither too superficial nor too deep. Typically, it is 0.5–1.0 cm below the skin. If necessary, small distal skin incisions assist in the creation of a loop. The graft is flushed with normal saline and any fat fragments removed from the lumen. The graft is cut obliquely such that the anastomosis is at least 1.5 times the diameter of the graft. Care must be taken to cut the graft to the correct length, avoiding both tension and excessive length leading to kinking. Vascular clamps are applied to the vessel (the venous anastomosis is usually performed first) and a venotomy of approximately 1.0–1.5 cm made using a no. 11 blade and Pott's scissors. The anastomosis is performed using a vascular suture such as 6/0 Prolene or Gore-Tex. On completion of the anastomosis, the suture is not tied. The arterial anastomosis is performed in a similar manner. Before releasing the vascular clamps, the graft is once again flushed with saline using an intravenous cannula (e.g. size 16 Abbocath or Wallace catheter), inserted through the venous anastomosis. A Watson–Cheyne dissector is used to dilate the vein proximally and distally as the vascular clamps are removed, and the suture is ligated. This procedure is repeated as the arterial clamps are removed and the suture ligated. If necessary, small swabs are applied to both anastomoses until haemostasis is secured. A palpable 'thrill' should be present along the length of the graft and in the draining vein proximally. The incisions are closed with chromic catgut to the fascia and nylon to the skin. Self-adhesive dressings are applied.

Postoperative care
Prophylactic broad-spectrum antibiotics should be given perioperatively and for 3 days postoperatively. Although the evidence is inconclusive, we recommend

administration of low-dose aspirin (e.g. 75 mg daily) long-term if there are no contraindications. Routine anticoagulation with warfarin is not indicated for most patients. Most patients can be mobilized within 24 hours even if the graft has been placed in the thigh.

Most patients develop some local bruising and swelling 24–72 hours postoperatively which may take at least 7–10 days to settle. Some grafts cause marked erythema during this time, which is not due to infection and settles spontaneously. While some manufacturers suggest that the graft can be used for dialysis within 3 or 4 days, it is normal practice to wait a minimum of 10–14 days. This allows good fibrous ingrowth to develop from surrounding tissues into the graft, minimizing bleeding problems after use, and also allows the bruising and swelling to settle.

Complications

Immediate surgical complications include bleeding and thrombosis. Their management is usually operative.

Long-term complications of PTFE grafts are similar to those of a standard AVF. Clotting, aneurysm formation and infection are more common than with an AVF. Infection in the presence of a graft – which is, after all, a foreign body – responds poorly to antibacterial therapy and demands surgical excision of the graft.

Graft thrombosis is usually associated with a stenosis at either the arterial or, more commonly, the venous anastomosis. This may be a technical complication or may follow the development of venous intimal neohyperplasia in the run-off vein close to or at the site of the venous anastomosis. In addition to thrombolysis or surgical thrombectomy, angiography is indicated to identify the underlying abnormality, which is likely to require correction.

Long-term solutions to the problem of intimal hyperplasia remain elusive. However, augmentation of the end of the graft to be attached to the vein may prove beneficial by enlarging the anastomosis and reducing shear stress on the wall of the effluent vein.

chapter 3

ACCESS FOR PERITONEAL DIALYSIS

This includes procedures for both temporary and long-term peritoneal dialysis.

TEMPORARY (RIGID) PERITONEAL DIALYSIS CATHETER INSERTION

Introduction
The indications for insertion of a temporary (hard) peritoneal catheter are limited. When urgent dialysis or fluid removal is required, haemofiltration, haemodialysis via a temporary vascular access or percutaneous placement of a soft peritoneal catheter may be the treatment of choice. Under circumstances where urgent treatment is required and these options do not exist or are inappropriate, placement of a hard temporary peritoneal catheter is justified. It is best avoided in patients destined for continuous ambulatory peritoneal dialysis in view of the associated increased risk of contamination of the peritoneal cavity with bacteria and/or potential damage to a viscus on insertion. Nevertheless, the procedure may be life-saving under appropriate circumstances.

Pre-procedure assessment
The abdomen should be inspected to ascertain whether previous operations have been carried out, whether an abdominal, inguinal or femoral hernia is present, and whether the bladder can be palpated or percussed. Previous surgery is associated with an increased risk of perforation of bowel adherent to the anterior abdominal wall. The risk of enlargement of or other complications associated with a hernia is increased by installation of dialysate into the peritoneal cavity. An enlarged bladder may be entered inadvertently by the catheter. If the bladder is full and the patient unable to empty it, urethral catheterization is necessary. The urethral catheter should be removed once drainage is complete. The patient should not be constipated – a pre-procedure laxative or enema may be required.

Equipment
A standard trochar and cannula set and connector are shown in Figure 3.1.

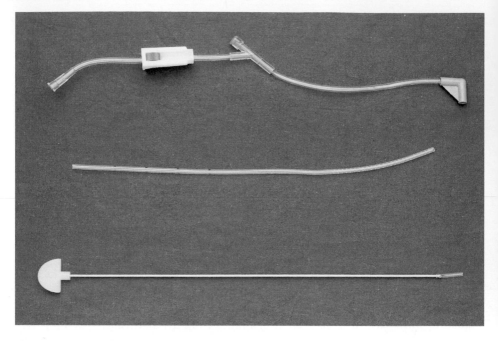

Figure 3.1 Standard trochar, cannula set and connector for temporary peritoneal dialysis.

Positioning of the patient
The patient should lie supine on one pillow.

Anaesthesia
Local anaesthesia with lignocaine 1 per cent without adrenaline should be employed.

Procedure
Shave the abdomen from the umbilicus to the pubis. Full aseptic precautions should thereafter be taken. Gown, mask and gloves are worn. Clean the skin with alcohol or iodine solution and wipe dry. Place surgical drapes. Inject lignocaine 1 per cent subcutaneously midway between umbilicus and pubis, then infiltrate local anaesthetic vertically downwards to the level of the linea alba. Allow 1–2 minutes for lignocaine to take effect. Remove trochar and cannula from the plastic envelope, and remove the trochar from the cannula. Inject 1–2 ml of heparin 1:1000 units down the catheter until heparin emanates from the small holes at the lower end of the catheter. This may reduce the risk of occlusion of the holes by fibrin plugs. Make a 1 cm vertical incision midway between the umbilicus and pubis, cutting down to the linea alba, which can be felt to grate against the scalpel blade. Re-insert the trochar into the cannula. Push the trochar and cannula vertically downwards until the peritoneal cavity is entered. It is helpful if the patient lifts his or her head off the pillow slightly

to tense the abdominal muscles immediately prior to inserting the catheter into the general peritoneal cavity. A distinct 'plop' is usually felt on entering the peritoneal cavity. Withdraw the trochar 2 cm or so from the end of the catheter and then push the assembled device gently downwards, aiming to position it in the pelvis on left or right sides.

When satisfactorily positioned, remove the trochar, leaving the catheter in place. Take care to exert gentle downward pressure on the catheter whilst removing the trochar in order to avoid extracting both together. With sterile scissors, trim the portion of the catheter above the abdominal skin to a length of approximately 3 cm. Run peritoneal dialysate through the giving set and connector, and connect up the effluent bag. Having run 500 ml of dialysate into the peritoneal cavity, cease to infuse dialysate into the peritoneal cavity and check that effluent drains freely from the peritoneal cavity. If it does so, obstruct effluent flow and resume dialysate flow until 2 litres of dialysate have been instilled. Insert a continuous suture around the cannula. Cut halfway through two gauze swabs and place them around the catheter exit site, the cut ends pointing in opposite directions. Tape the catheter in place, ensuring that it is not kinked.

Post-procedure care

A meticulous aseptic technique is required by nursing and other staff when setting up fresh dialysate bags. Application of povidone iodine to the catheter exit site every few days may be of value in preventing exit site infection and peritonitis.

Failure of dialysate to flow into the peritoneal cavity may occur if the tip of the catheter is wedged against the wall of the pelvis or bowel. Conversely, dialysate may flow in readily but fail to drain under these circumstances. Failure of dialysate drainage may result from displacement of the catheter from the pelvis (Figures 3.2 and 3.3). At times a plug of fibrin appears to exert a ball-valve effect at the tip of the catheter, allowing dialysate to flow in but not out of the peritoneal cavity. Later failure of drainage may result from the omentum becoming wrapped around the catheter. Poor flows and subcutaneous abdominal oedema indicate that a portion of the catheter lies outside the peritoneal cavity.

Entry of the catheter into the bladder should not occur if adequate precautions are taken (see above). If this does occur, the diagnosis is readily made as the patient will void large quantities of dialysate per urethram. If doubt exists about whether dialysate or urine is being voided, 'stix' testing for glucose should resolve the matter, a strongly positive result indicating the presence of dialysate. If the bladder has been entered, urethral catheter drainage for 2–3 weeks may allow sealing of the defect, failing which open surgery may be required. Entry of the catheter into the bowel and bowel perforation demand that a surgical opinion be obtained and laparotomy will normally be necessary.

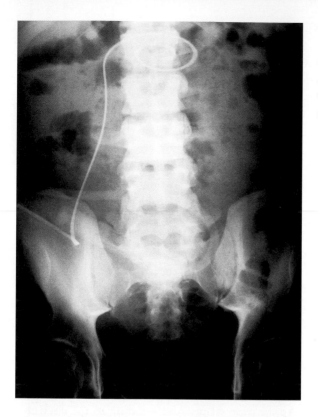

Figure 3.2 Peritoneal catheter tip (in this case a soft Tenckhoff catheter) lying in the upper abdomen rather than in the pelvis, with consequent failure of effluent drainage.

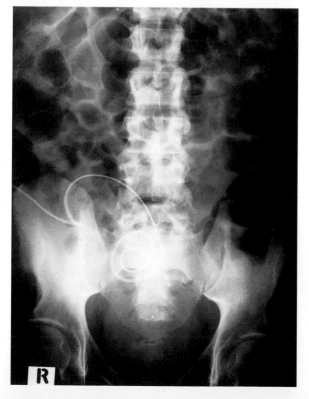

Figure 3.3 Peritoneal catheter in an ideal position.

LONG-TERM (SOFT) PERITONEAL DIALYSIS CATHETER INSERTION

Insertion of soft peritoneal catheters can be carried out either percutaneously or by formal surgery.

PERCUTANEOUS INSERTION OF SOFT PERITONEAL CATHETERS

Introduction
This is a technique for insertion of soft peritoneal catheters for continuous ambulatory peritoneal dialysis (CAPD) or automated peritoneal dialysis (APD). It employs catheters with a peel-away sheath, placed into the peritoneal cavity via a guide-wire. The principle is the same as that employed for insertion of central venous catheters (Chapter 2). The procedure is generally performed under local anaesthesia with intravenous sedation. It can be performed outside a full operating theatre environment but it is advantageous to have X-ray screening available to confirm the positions of the guide-wire and catheter. Strict aseptic precautions are mandatory. Both straight and curled catheters may be inserted in this way. Most patients will have opted for long-term peritoneal dialysis treatment of end-stage renal failure.

The main contraindication to the procedure is previous abdominal surgery, particularly involving the lower abdomen and pelvis. The presence of known adhesions below the level of the umbilicus should be considered an absolute contraindication to percutaneous catheter insertion and an open catheter insertion method should be adopted instead. In general, the technique is used to insert a first catheter into a largely or entirely 'virgin' abdomen.

Preoperative assessment
This is as set out on p. 45.

Equipment
This is shown in Figure 3.4. It comprises:

- A straight or curled catheter
- Peel-away sheath and dilator
- Guide-wire
- Introducer needle
- Catheter stylette
- Tunnelling tool
- Catheter connector
- A scalpel (no. 11 or 15)
- Skin sutures (such as 3/0 nylon), local anaesthetic, normal saline, syringes and needles, adhesive dressings and skin disinfectant (usually aqueous povidone iodine solution).

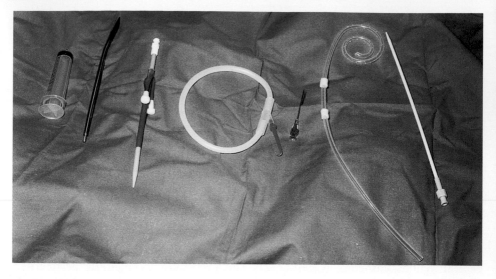

Figure 3.4 Equipment for insertion of a soft peritoneal catheter.

Positioning and preparation of the patient

The patient lies supine upon a bed or operating table, support for the head being provided by a single pillow. The patient should not be constipated (a pre-procedure laxative or enema may be required if this is the case). If the bladder is palpable or percussible, it must be emptied prior to the procedure, catheterization being carried out if necessary.

Anaesthesia

Anaesthesia is with 1 per cent lignocaine without adrenaline supplemented by intravenous sedation as required.

Procedure

Shave the abdomen from the umbilicus to the pubis. Mark the skin (with magic marker) at the approximate position of the catheter exit site. Thereafter, full aseptic precautions should be taken. Prepare the skin with alcohol or povidone iodine and drape with sterile towels. Anaesthetize the skin approximately midway between the umbilicus and the pubis with 1 per cent lignocaine without adrenaline. Make a transverse skin incision and dissect down to the rectus sheath with dissecting forceps. Inject local anaesthetic into deeper structures. Puncture the peritoneum with the introducer needle and advance the guide-wire gently into the right or left pelvis (Figure 3.5). Then remove the introducer needle and insert the peel-away sheath and dilator along the guide-wire into the peritoneal cavity. Remove the guide-wire and dilator, and place the peritoneal catheter over the stylette. Introduce the catheter and stylette into the peritoneal cavity via the sheath, and then peel the sheath away leaving the catheter *in situ*. Withdraw the catheter stylette. Check that the catheter is patent by instilling

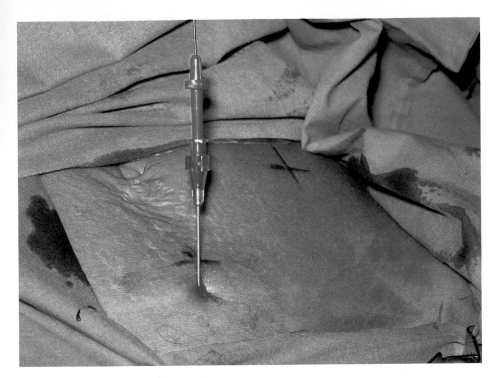

Figure 3.5 Guide-wire being advanced during the procedure for insertion of a soft peritoneal catheter.

50 ml warm normal saline through it. Ensure that the inner cuff of the dual-cuff catheter lies within the rectus sheath. Anaesthetize the catheter exit site with 1 per cent lignocaine without adrenaline and fashion the exit site with a stab incision using a no. 11 scalpel blade. The exit site should lie approximately 2 cm beyond the outer cuff of the catheter. Draw the catheter through a subcutaneous skin tunnel using a tunnelling tool. Attach the connector and retest the catheter by infusion of a further 50 ml of warm saline. If doubt exists about whether satisfactory flow will be obtained, a 1 litre dialysate exchange can be performed at this stage to define the situation. Apply the closure cap, apply interrupted sutures to the skin, and then apply gauze dressings and secure the catheter with adhesive tape (Figure 3.6).

Useful tips
- Confirm the introducer needle is in the peritoneum using contrast X-ray screening.
- Use X-ray guidance for the guide-wire and catheter (Figure 3.3).
- Rinse the CAPD catheter in normal saline and soak Dacron cuffs thoroughly.
- Utilize any natural bias in the catheter to improve stability.
- Place a purse-string absorbable suture into the rectus sheath to reduce risk of leakage.

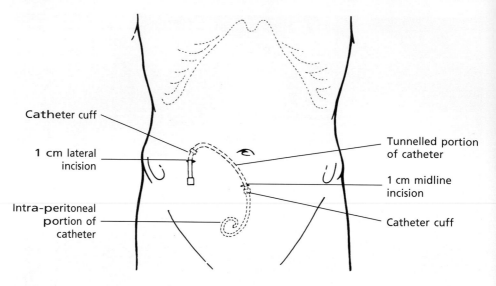

Figure 3.6 Percutaneously inserted soft peritoneal catheter in place.

Postoperative care

Adequate analgesia must be provided. The patient should be observed for signs of bleeding or bowel perforation. Ideally, no dialysate exchanges should be carried out for several days after catheter placement. It is important that the catheter be immobilized by the dressings. Skin sutures are removed on the 10th postoperative day.

Complications

Flow failure
Causes:

- Constipation
- Catheter migration
- Omental occlusion
- Clot/fibrin occlusion
- Early peritonitis
- Kinked catheter
- Blocked or defective dialysate lines or catheter connector
- Placement outside the peritoneum.

Management:

- Check dialysate lines
- Plain abdominal radiograph
- Treat constipation
- Instil thrombolytic agent (urokinase 25 000 units)
- Surgical exploration.

Dialysate leakage
External
External leakage results in peritoneal dialysate leaking through the abdominal wall puncture, tracking along the subcutaneous tunnel, and leaking from the exit site. The diagnosis is usually very obvious but can be confirmed by measuring the glucose concentration of the escaping fluid with a reagent strip. A strongly positive result confirms the fluid is dialysate.
Internal
Escape of dialysate into extraperitoneal structures can present in a variety of ways, including:

- Abdominal wall oedema
- Perineal/scrotal oedema (Figure 3.7a)
- Pleural effusion (sometimes associated with a congenital diaphragmatic defect)
- Unexplained poor drainage.

It can be associated with a groin hernia or persistent processus vaginalis (Figure 3.7b).

The precise site of leakage can be located using intraperitoneal contrast media combined with plain radiography or computed tomography scanning.
Management
Minor leaks may respond to a reduction in exchange volume, but the preferred approach is to suspend dialysis and leave the peritoneum dry. There is no established optimum duration of rest but, in general, a week is usually enough, although more major leaks may require up to 2 weeks to resolve.

Recurrent leaks, especially those associated with abdominal wall defects, may require surgical intervention or abandonment of peritoneal dialysis.

Bleeding
Intraperitoneal
This usually stops spontaneously, and therefore demands no specific action. However, in severe cases, surgical intervention may be necessary.
Exit site
Local pressure may suffice. Recurrent bleeding can be managed by placing a haemostatic purse-string suture around the exit site. Care must be taken to avoid damage to the catheter, and the suture should be removed at the earliest opportunity as it represents an exit-site infection hazard.

Wound
Again, the initial approach should be to apply local pressure, but additional interrupted skin sutures may be required.

Perforation of abdominal organs
This is a serious complication and involves perforation of the large bowel, small bowel or bladder. Surgical intervention is required in the form of an exploratory

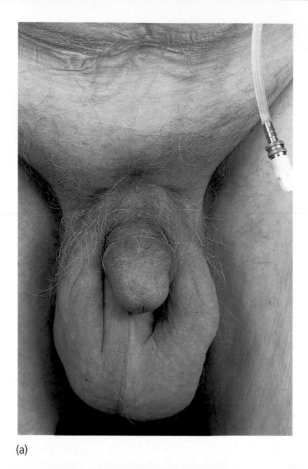

(a)

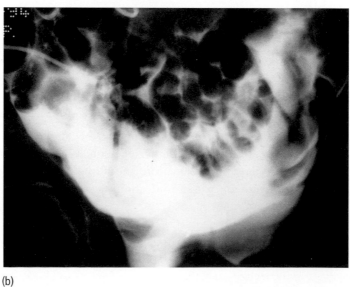

(b)

Figure 3.7 (a) Scrotal oedema caused by leakage of dialysate via a persistent processus vaginalis. **(b)** Peritoneogram showing persistent processus vaginalis.

laparotomy for bowel perforation and in some cases a defunctioning procedure is indicated. If the bladder has been entered, urethral catheter drainage for 2–3 weeks may allow sealing of the defect, failing which open surgery may be required.

SURGICAL INSERTION OF SOFT PERITONEAL CATHETERS

Indications
In some centres, open operation is the standard procedure for all patients. However, if the percutaneous technique is available, open operation is reserved for those with a history of previous abdominal surgery or CAPD-related peritonitis, in view of the likely presence of intraperitonal adhesions or adhesion of bowel to the anterior abdominal wall.

Preoperative assessment
It is essential to examine the patient carefully to exclude any abdominal hernias. If present, these should be repaired prior to commencing CAPD, although it may be appropriate to perform the hernia repair and catheter insertion under the same anaesthetic. Routine investigations to prepare the patient for a general anaesthetic are required. In discussion with the patient and nursing staff, the preferred exit site should be defined and marked as previously described, to allow comfortable use and minimize irritation from clothing.

Equipment
The catheters employed are described earlier in this chapter.

Positioning the patient
The procedure is performed in the operating theatre with full sterile precautions. The patient lies supine on the operating table.

Anaesthesia
The operation may be performed using local, regional or general anaesthesia. In most patients, general anaesthesia with full muscle relaxation is the preferred option. Spinal or epidural anaesthesia are acceptable alternatives, but local anaesthesia is rarely appropriate even when combined with intravenous sedation.

Procedure
The abdomen is cleaned with antiseptic skin preparation and draped. The favoured incision is a right or left gridiron incision approximately half way along a line from the anterior superior iliac crest to the umbilicus. However, it is preferable to avoid previous incisions and therefore, if necessary, a sub-umbilical midline incision may be used. A 2–3 cm opening is made in the peritoneum and the abdominal cavity explored with a finger to establish the presence and extent of any adhesions. In particular, the pelvis should be examined – exten-

sive pelvic adhesions are likely to render CAPD unsuccessful. During this initial exploration of the abdominal cavity it is also valuable to assess the position and mobility of the omentum. It is not necessary to remove the omentum routinely, but if it is relatively free and mobile a limited omentectomy is indicated to reduce the likelihood that the catheter will become wrapped in omentum.

The technique using a twin-cuff catheter is described, although claims have been made that a single-cuff catheter gives equally good results. Using a long pair of forceps, the end of the catheter is passed into the pelvis, lying anterior to the rectum but behind the bladder (and uterus in a female). In most patients, correct positioning of the end of the catheter results in the first Dacron cuff of the catheter lying at the level of the peritoneal opening. With the first Dacron cuff lying superficial to it, the peritoneum is sutured with chromic catgut until it is closed tightly around the catheter. Gentle traction on the catheter then allows two or three sutures to be taken through both peritoneum and the cuff, to produce a secure peritoneal closure. Free flow of saline into and out of the peritoneum is checked at this stage. Using a tunnelling device, the catheter is brought through a subcutaneous tunnel to the previously chosen exit site (Figure 3.8). It is essential that the second Dacron cuff, lying subcutaneously, is at least 2 cm away from the exit site. Free flow of saline is confirmed, 5 ml of heparin (1000 units/ml) are instilled into the catheter and the appropriate connector and cap are fitted. The muscle layers of the wound are closed with Vicryl and the skin sutured with interrupted nylon. Adhesive dressings are applied over the incision and, separately, over the catheter and exit site. No stitching should be used to secure the catheter; it is not necessary and encourages exit-site infection.

Postoperative care
This is described earlier in the chapter.

Complications
The complications of CAPD relevant to the surgeon are listed below.

Fluid leak
This presents typically as fluid leaking around the catheter when fluid exchanges commence. The management is normally conservative – cessation of peritoneal dialysis for 10–14 days usually allows adequate healing to occur. If the leak persists after an adequate rest period, it is likely that the catheter will require removal and re-insertion.

Fluid extravasation
This may occur at any time – possibly after months or years of uncomplicated peritoneal dialysis. Fluid leaks into the tissues of the anterior abdominal wall producing oedema, discoloration and discomfort. As with an early leak, the management is initially conservative – cessation of dialysis for 10–14 days – followed by replacement of the catheter if the problem persists.

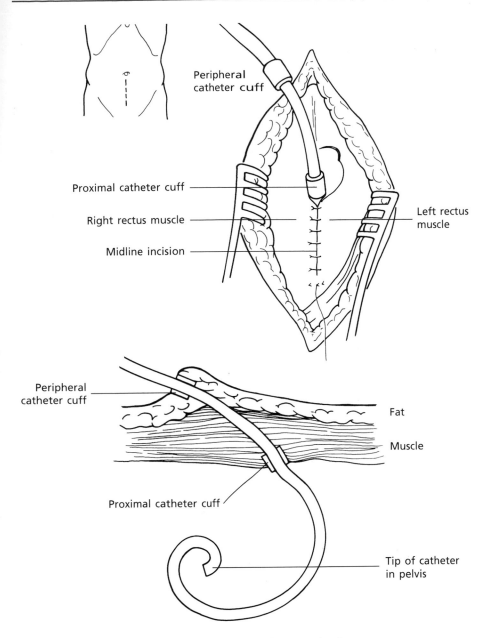

Figure 3.8 Open surgical placement of twin-cuff soft peritoneal catheter.

Patent processus vaginalis

An undetected, asymptomatic patent processus vaginalis (in the absence of an inguinal hernia) will allow peritoneal fluid to leak into the scrotum (Figure 3.7a). Presentation is with sudden scrotal swelling which may occur at the start of dialysis or at any time thereafter. Cessation of dialysis leads to rapid resolution of the swelling but surgical repair is required before peritoneal dialysis is restarted. The history and examination, surprisingly, do not always allow a firm diagnosis of the size of the problem, in which case a small volume of radio-opaque contrast introduced through the peritoneal catheter into the peritoneum will demonstrate which side requires operation.

Failure of inflow and/or outflow of dialysate fluid

Intraperitoneal adhesions, noted at the time of catheter insertion, may prevent successful exchanges. Normally fluid will drain neither in nor out. No effective treatment is available. Transfer to haemodialysis is required.

One-way obstruction, i.e. fluid will drain into the peritoneal cavity but not out, is often the result of the omentum becoming wrapped around the catheter. Less commonly, loops of small bowel or even a large 'floppy' bladder may produce the same problem. Free flow is also less likely if the tip of the catheter moves out of the pelvis and lies elsewhere within the abdominal cavity. Constipation may mimic all the above and, before embarking on intervention, it is important to ensure that the bowel is not loaded.

Surgery may be required to relieve one-way obstruction. Ideally, the peritoneum is opened through a small separate incision, e.g. a lower midline incision, which allows 'watertight' peritoneal closure and thus immediate postoperative recommencement of peritoneal dialysis. The operative procedure will depend on the findings but usually involves either simple flushing and repositioning of the catheter or limited omentectomy.

Infection

A detailed description of the treatment of CAPD-associated infection is outside the scope of this book.

Infection may be:

- Unresolved acute peritonitis. The catheter should be removed.
- Recurrent peritonitis with the identical infective agent (relapsing peritonitis). This suggests colonization of the catheter, which should be removed.
- Infection in the subcutaneous tunnel. This may respond to antibiotic therapy but removal of the catheter is often required.
- Exit-site infection. This may be chronic and trivial, which may perhaps be ignored, or severe. Antibiotic therapy may be successful, but catheter removal may become necessary.

Extruded cuff

The second cuff, which lies in the subcutaneous tunnel, may extrude through the exit site. Replacement of the catheter with a new one is usually carried out.

REMOVAL OF SOFT PERITONEAL CATHETERS

This may be performed surgically or by traction on the catheter using intravenous sedation or general anaesthesia. Traction must not be used if the CAPD catheter is designed with 'flanges' at the intraperitoneal tip because there is a serious risk of damage to the bowel. If the catheter breaks during an attempt to remove it by traction, it is essential to re-operate to remove the retained portion. On occasions, the catheter is pulled free from one or both of the Dacron cuffs that remain *in situ*, usually in the subcutaneous tissues. Surgical removal is required, as there is a significant risk of subsequent sepsis.

chapter 4

RENAL BIOPSY

Introduction

Renal biopsy is indicated if an exact histological diagnosis may influence management in a beneficial way or provide a necessary prognosis. Since the procedure carries morbidity, a small risk of haemorrhage demanding intervention, including nephrectomy, and since there is an associated mortality (approximately 1 in 1500), biopsy is not justifiable solely for research purposes or curiosity as to the diagnosis alone. Biopsy is not needed when the diagnosis is almost certain on clinical grounds, e.g. in Type 1 diabetes with non-renal complications, such as proliferative retinopathy and no clinical or laboratory suspicion of alternative aetiology; shortly after beta-haemolytic streptococcal infection; or after relevant drug therapy, e.g. pencillamine.

Recognized indications in adults include:

- Nephrotic syndrome.
- Unexplained renal impairment with normal or near normal kidney size.
- Failure to recover from apparent acute renal failure.
- Suspicion of systemic vasculitis/crescentic glomerulonephritis.
- Biopsy of a poorly functioning transplant kidney, if the differential diagnosis between rejection, acute tubular necrosis, immunosuppressive drug nephrotoxicity, or drug-induced or infective interstitial nephritis is in doubt.

Asymptomatic proteinuria of modest degree with no impairment of glomerular filtration rate, and in the absence of hypoproteinaemia, and isolated microscopic haematuria are not normally considered indications for biopsy.

Contraindications include:

- Haemorrhagic diathesis which cannot be corrected.
- Small kidneys.
- Single kidney (transplant kidney and a single kidney with chronically very poor function are exceptions to this rule, the latter because haemorrhage with consequent nephrectomy would have less disastrous consequences than if the kidney were to be functioning well).
- Uncontrolled hypertension and/or uraemia.
- Gross obesity.
- Non-compliant patient.
- Where the diagnosis is obvious on anatomical grounds, e.g. reflux nephropathy, polycystic kidneys, urinary tract obstruction.
- Severe anaemia (haemoglobin less than 8 g/dl prior to correction).

Pre-procedure assessment

The patient should be given a written account of the procedure and should be told of the risks of bleeding (10 per cent risk of macroscopic haematuria; 1 in 500 prospect of severe haemorrhage requiring transfusion/intervention by renal angiography with infusion of anticoagulant, sclerosant and/or insertion of arterial blocking device; 1 in 750 prospect of nephrectomy; 1 in 1500 mortality). The patient should also be warned that there may be some discomfort over the flank or shoulder tip on the side of the biopsy following the procedure.

Preliminary investigations

- Haemoglobin concentration.
- Prothrombin time, platelet count, partial thromboplastin time with kaolin, bleeding time (to be less than 8 minutes).
- Blood group testing and saving of serum for cross-match.

Correct any coagulation abnormalities detected, e.g. by infusion of platelets or fresh frozen plasma. Provided coronary artery disease is not suspected or known to be present, we recommend that desmopressin (DDAVP) 20 µg in 100 ml normal saline be infused intravenously during the 30 minutes before biopsy if serum creatinine exceeds 300 µmol/l in view of the impaired platelet function that accompanies severe renal failure.

Equipment

Alcohol or iodine solution, gauze swabs, lignocaine 1 per cent (10–20 ml), green needle, orange needle, 22 G lumbar puncture needle, Trucut biopsy needle (Figure 4.1) size 14 or 18 G (a 14 G Trucut is usually employed for native kidney biopsy and an 18 G needle for transplant biopsy), Biopty gun (Bard) (if to be used) (Figure 4.2), 10 ml syringe, orange stick, gown, mask, gloves, surgical drapes, firm pillow, firm mattress or board under bed. Ten per cent formal saline or phosphate-buffered saline solution.

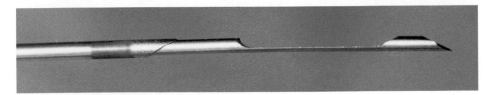

Figure 4.1 Trucut renal biopsy needle.

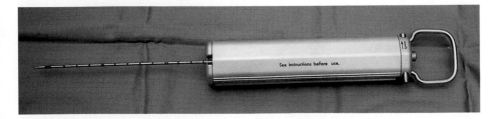

Figure 4.2 Biopty gun for renal biopsy.

NATIVE RENAL BIOPSY

Positioning the patient

The patient lies prone with a bolster or pillow under the abdomen and the head turned to the right side. It is essential to ensure that the patient is parallel to the bed or operating table rather than in a curved position, and comfortable so that the position can be maintained throughout the procedure. If the patient moves, so will the position of the kidney to be biopsied. The patient should practise holding his or her breath in inspiration for a few seconds on command as this will be required during the biopsy procedure. If respiration continues while the biopsy is being taken, the kidney will present a moving target. An adequate specimen may not be obtained and the risk of renal damage is increased.

Anaesthesia is with lignocaine without adrenaline; 10 ml of 1 per cent lignocaine is usually adequate, but if the patient is large or the kidney is deep, 15–20 ml may be required.

Procedure (without Biopty gun)

Locate the position and depth of the kidney by ultrasound (Figure 4.3) using a 3.5 MHz transducer and with the patient's breath held in inspiration. The lower pole of the kidney is identified and a mark is made on the skin, corresponding to the lower pole. The ultrasound image is frozen and the depth of the posterior margin of the lower pole from the skin surface is measured on the image.

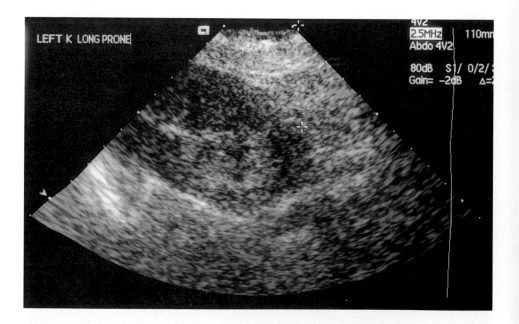

Figure 4.3 Use of ultrasound to locate the kidney to be biopsied and its depth from the skin surface.

The left kidney is more conveniently biopsied than the right by a right-handed operator. Sterile precautions are taken from this point onwards. Hands should be washed, and sterile gown, mask and gloves should be worn.

Swab the skin generously with alcohol or iodine, and apply drapes. Inject local anaesthetic subcutaneously at the biopsy point on the skin using an orange needle. With the patient holding his or her breath in inspiration, inject lignocaine vertically downwards via a green needle until resistance is felt from the capsule of the kidney. In addition, infuse lignocaine at an angle of 15 degrees to the vertical. Allow 1–2 minutes for the local anaesthetic to take effect, then insert a lumbar puncture needle at an angle of 15 degrees down the track until resistance is felt from the lower pole of the kidney. Inject more local anaesthetic. Check the ultrasound measurement of the depth of the kidney by aligning the orange stick with the lumbar puncture needle, breaking it at the top of the shaft of the needle and measuring the difference between the length of the stick and that of the needle after its removal. Advance the Trucut needle perpendicularly or at a slight angle (not more than 15 degrees) along the track to the required depth (Figure 4.4). In each case, advance the Trucut with the patient holding his or her breath in inspiration. Periodically, ask the patient to breathe in and out to see if the characteristic swing of the Trucut needle occurs, indicating that it is within the lower pole of the kidney. When the Trucut needle is just adjacent to or within the lower pole, ask the patient to hold his or her breath in inspiration and take the biopsy by sharply depressing the head of the trochar portion of the Trucut needle at the same time ensuring that the shaft is not withdrawn (the right hand is used to depress and the left to advance the shaft over the tip of the trochar, thus securing the biopsy material). Then

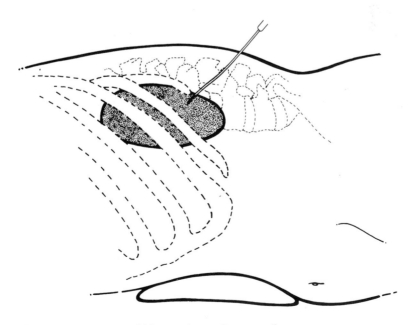

Figure 4.4 Transcutaneous renal biopsy using a Trucut needle.

withdraw the Trucut as a whole. Press on the biopsy exit site with a gauze swab.

Push the trochar down and out of the cannula of the Trucut into the liquid solution to be used in order to examine the biopsy specimen. If the biopsy floats, perinephric fat alone may have been obtained. If no satisfactory specimen has been obtained, a second biopsy may be attempted. No more than three passes with entry into the kidney should be attempted. If the biopsy is placed into 10 per cent formol saline, this allows examination by light microscopy, electron microscopy and immunoperoxidase staining. Alternatively, the specimen may be placed into phosphate-buffered saline, then examined under a dissecting microscope. A portion containing glomeruli is then cut off with a scalpel blade and placed into gluteraldehyde solution. This gives better results from electron microscopy. The remaining specimen is placed into 10 per cent formal saline. Apply a pressure dressing to the biopsy exit site with gauze. Return the patient to the ward.

Procedure employing an automated spring-loaded needle or gun (Biopty gun)

The technique using the Biopty gun (a spring-loaded device which holds a modified Trucut needle) differs from the above for a number of reasons. The needle, held in the gun, is guided to the renal margin using ultrasound visualization. Because the needle is held in the heavy gun, needle swing cannot be elicited. This technique requires considerably greater ultrasound scanning skills than biopsy without use of semi-automated devices.

The Trucut needle is inserted into the gun and the safety lock applied. Once the needle has been advanced to the correct position, the safety lock is taken off and the gun fired by pressing on the button at the top of the gun. The usual throw (or movement of the needle into the tissues) with a standard gun is 2.3 cm. More recently developed alternatives to the Biopty gun are a variety of disposable spring-loaded needles, e.g. Temno needle (Bauer). These have a spring-loaded cocking device in the handle which is cocked before the needle is advanced.

Scans are made over the skin of the back with a 3.5 MHz transducer and the patient's breath held in inspiration. The lower pole of the kidney is identified and a skin mark is made over the mid-lower pole. The ultrasound image is frozen and the depth of the posterior margin of the lower pole from the skin is measured on the image. Local anaesthetic is infiltrated from the skin mark to the posterior renal margin using a 22 G spinal needle and ultrasound visualization during suspended inspiration. The Trucut needle in the Biopty gun is then held in the right hand and advanced to the posterior renal margin, again during suspended inspiration and with ultrasound visualization, using the transducer held in the left hand (Figure 4.5). It is often difficult to see the tip of the spinal and biopsy needles. Their position is identified by making small to and fro needle movements. These cause movements of the soft tissues, which can be visualized. A depth measurement taken previously from the posterior lower renal pole may also be used to help correct positioning of the needle by marking

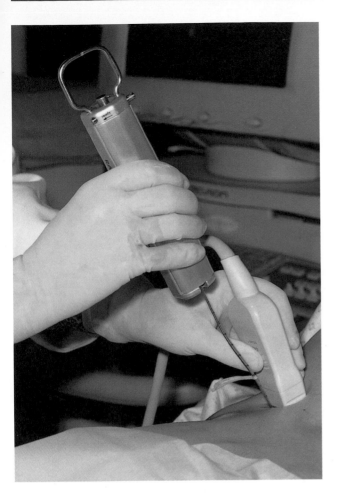

Figure 4.5 Transcutaneous renal biopsy using a Biopty gun.

the measurement of the needle with a 'Steristrip', or by using the centimetre markers on the needle.

When the needle tip is in the correct position, the Biopty gun is fired while the patient holds his or her breath in inspiration. Normally, the operator does not scan whilst firing the gun. The gun rapidly advances the Trucut into the kidney and cuts the specimen. The needle is then withdrawn in the gun. Once the needle has been removed from the gun, the renal specimen is retrieved from the notch and placed in fixative as described previously. If a satisfactory specimen is not obtained, two further passes may be made.

Post-procedure care:

- The patient rests supine in bed (except for using the lavatory) for 24 hours.
- Pulse and blood pressure are taken every 15 minutes for 4 hours, half-hourly for 4 hours and hourly thereafter following biopsy until 24 hours has elapsed.
- Hypotension or tachycardia (blood pressure fall greater than 20 mmHg systolic or diastolic from pre-biopsy state, or pulse rate over 100

beats/minute) or other suspicion of haemorrhage requires the immediate attention of medical staff.

- The patient leaves hospital 24 hours after the procedure providing no complications have occurred.
- The patient is warned to avoid heavy lifting, gardening, etc. for 2 weeks.

TRANSPLANT RENAL BIOPSY

The technique for transplant biopsy (Figure 4.6) is simpler because the kidney is usually quite superficial in the iliac fossa. Preprocedure assessment is similar to that described on p. 61, modified as appropriate to the different anatomical position of the kidney to be biopsied.

Biopsies may be obtained from either pole, whichever is more accessible, with the patient supine. Ultrasound scanning is used to localize the appropriate pole and measure its depth from the skin surface. After infiltration of local anaesthetic, either the needle is advanced to this depth or the needle is visualized using ultrasound as it is passed to the renal margin. An 18 G Trucut usually yields an adequate specimen. A hand-held or automated needle (or needle in a gun) may be used. No more than three passes should be made. The kidney does not move with respiration, so the patient can breathe quietly during the procedure. Direct pressure on the biopsy exit site for 5 minutes may be used to exert pressure on the relatively superficial transplant kidney following the procedure. If appropriate, the patient may leave hospital a few hours after the procedure.

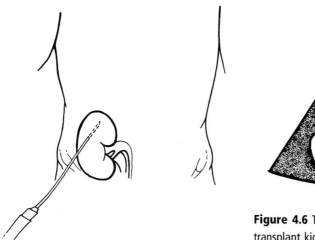

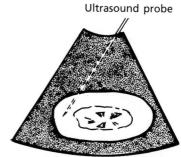

Ultrasound probe

Figure 4.6 Transcutaneous biopsy of a transplant kidney. Note – in contrast to the native kidney biopsy – that the lower pole of the transplant kidney is *not* aimed for.

chapter 5

BONE BIOPSY

Introduction

Abnormalities in mineral metabolism complicating impaired renal function regularly lead to clinically significant bone disease. The development of satisfactory assays for parathyroid hormone and biochemical markers of bone turnover have improved the clinician's ability to diagnose and monitor renal osteodystrophy. Bone histology remains, however, the diagnostic 'gold standard' and is invaluable when symptomatic bone disease presents a diagnostic problem. Bone biopsy remains an essential component of metabolic bone disease research.

Tetracycline is deposited in bone at sites of osteoid mineralization. Two short separated courses of oral tetracycline double-label the bone, providing information on the extent and rate of mineralization, and the rate of osteoid production. This allows a distinction to be made between impaired mineralization of osteoid produced at a normal rate (e.g. osteomalacia) and normal mineralization in the face of excessively rapid production of osteoid (e.g. Paget's disease of bone). The following labelling regimen may be used in adult dialysis patients providing there is no history of tetracycline allergy and advice is given regarding photosensitivity and other side-effects:

- Tetracycline 250 mg twice daily on days 1–4 inclusive.
- Demeclocycline 150 mg twice daily on days 15–19 inclusive.
- Bone biopsy on day 23 or 24.

Histomorphometry and tetracycline-labelling provide both quantitative and dynamic information to supplement histological interpretation of bone biopsies.

Preoperative assessment

A full blood count and clotting screen should be performed prior to biopsy. Haemodialysis patients should be biopsied on a non-dialysis day (since heparin is used to anticoagulate the extracorporeal circuit) and heparin administration should be minimized for 1–2 weeks after biopsy.

Equipment

A standard bone biopsy set consists of an inner and outer trephine, trochar and rod used to expel the core of bone from the inner trephine. An alternative approach is to use a bone biopsy 'gun' (Figure 5.1).

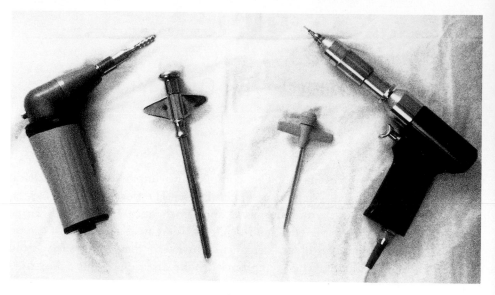

Figure 5.1 Bone biopsy equipment.

Positioning the patient

The patient is placed in a dorsi-recumbent position on a firm operating table. The iliac crest is the preferred site for bone biopsy carried out to investigate metabolic bone disease. Rib biopsy frequently results in fracture and the large diameter of the biopsy needle precludes the use of the sternum for biopsy. The pelvis is positioned to bring the biopsy site towards the operator and is raised 5–10 cm above the operating table using a sandbag under the ipsilateral buttock. Slight flexion of the ipsilateral knee and external rotation of the foot relaxes the muscles covering the biopsy site.

Anaesthesia

This is with 10–20 ml of 1 per cent lignocaine without adrenaline, usually combined with an intramuscular opiate and anti-emetic administered half an hour before the procedure. Intravenous sedation immediately before the procedure will be appropriate in selected patients. In sedated patients, respiratory and cardiovascular status should be monitored.

Procedure

The procedure should ideally be carried out in an operating theatre. The skin overlying the biopsy site, 2 cm below and behind the anterior superior iliac spine is sterilized with alcohol or an iodine solution. The surrounding area is then covered with sterile towelling, leaving the biopsy site exposed. The skin and subcutaneous tissues are infiltrated with 10–20 ml of 1 per cent lignocaine via a syringe and needle. The needle is then cautiously advanced to the periosteum and, when the resistance of bone is felt, the periosteum and subperiosteal regions are carefully infiltrated. Once local anaesthesia is achieved, a 2 cm skin incision is made and extended down to the periosteum. Soft-tissue haemorrhage is controlled through compression by surgical swabs. The trochar is placed into the outer trephine and introduced into the incision perpendicular to the surface of the ilium. Both are advanced to the surface of the bone. The outer trephine is firmly pressed into the periosteum, forcing the teeth of the trephine to cut in and obtain a secure purchase on the surface of the bone. The trochar is then removed and replaced by the inner trephine. An assistant should apply appropriate counterpressure against the contralateral pelvic wall as the biopsy is performed. The inner trephine is firmly rotated, allowing the teeth to cut through the bone until the ilium is completely penetrated to provide a sample with an inner and outer cortex. The inner trephine is gently rotated without inward pressure to detach fibrous tissue adherent to the inner surface of the specimen. The inner and outer trephine are removed together using a gentle rocking motion.

Haemostasis is secured through local compression with surgical swabs. The skin is closed with interrupted silk or nylon sutures and a dry, transparent dressing applied. The towels and sandbag are removed and the patient is repositioned to lie on the biopsy site for approximately 2 hours to ensure optimum haemostasis. Blood pressure and pulse should be monitored every 15 minutes for 1 hour, half-hourly for 1 hour, then hourly for 3 hours.

The specimen is removed gently from the inner trephine by the use of the expelling rod. The specimen should be placed in 70–100 per cent ethanol for transportation to the laboratory. Formalin should not be employed because this may leach tetracycline and aluminium from the bone. A 10 per cent phosphate-buffered formalin solution may, however, be used as a fixative for non-tetracycline-labelled specimens and for patients in whom aluminium deposition in bone is not suspected.

As an alternative, the biopsy may be taken using an electrically driven biopsy gun.

Post-biopsy care

Unless a general anaesthetic has been employed, the patient may return home 4–6 hours after the biopsy, having been advised to rest and to avoid driving a vehicle for at least 24 hours. The patient should be advised to seek medical advice if the wound becomes painful or reddened, or if a discharge develops. The wound should be inspected after 7 days and the stitches removed 7–10 days after the biopsy.

Complications

The majority of patients report moderate discomfort as the local anaesthetic agent wears off. The use of a 100 mg diclofenac suppository provides excellent analgesia, with patients only occasionally requiring supplementary oral analgesia for the first postoperative night. Extensive bruising and bleeding from the biopsy site may occur but this is uncommon. Wound infection is rare; if it does occur, skin sutures should be removed and appropriate antibacterial therapy administered.

INDEX

Page numbers printed in **bold** type refer to **figures**; those in *italic* to tables.

NEPHROLOGY

Edited by:
R. Jamison, Stanford University, USA
R. Wilkinson, Freeman Hospital, UK

Nephrology has been produced by an international team of authorities who have selected the most important aspects of renal disease to create a manageable accessible volume. A wide perspective on current research findings is offered along with an understanding of the disease and its impact on practical patient management. Clear layout and design, with good use of colour make this a user-friendly and appealing book that will be of real practical value to all physicians dealing with renal disease.

Key Features
- Concentrates on common conditions
- Emphasises practical everyday issues
- Over 500 illustrations
- Essential information in a single volume

Contents
Normal structure and function/ Structure/ Renal physiology/ Renal regulation and volume composition of body fluids/ Blood pressure and function/ Renal biology/ Impaired renal function/ Methods of assessment/ Fluid and electrolyte disorders/ Other disorders secondary to kidney disease/ Diseases of the kidney and their treatment/ Inherited and developmental diseases/ Diseases of the kidney in pregnancy/ Systematic diseases and renal involvement/ Primary diseases in the glomerulus/ Diseases of renal interstitium/ Other diseases/ General management of chronic renal diseases/ General management principles/ Dialysis and related procedures/ Transplantation.

1998	HB	1172pp	391 b/w & 126 col illus	ISBN 0 412 60930 4	£145.00

Diagnostic Tests in Nephrology

Edited by:
J. Bradley & K. Smith
Addenbrooke's Hospital, Cambridge, UK

Diagnostic Tests in Nephrology brings together for the first time detailed practical guidance on the full range of evaluative procedures available for the investigation of renal disease.

Key Features
- Thorough review of diagnostic tests for patients with renal disease
- A clear two-colour presentation making information easily accessible
- Discusses the interpretation of abnormal results
- Essential information in a single volume

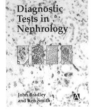

Contents
Part One: Diagnostic tests/ Biochemistry/ Haematology/ Urinalysis/ Immunology/ Radiology/ Nuclear medicine/ Renal biopsy/ Genetics **Part Two**: Renal investigations in clinical practice/ Acute renal failure/ Chronic renal failure/ Transplantation/ Hypertension/ Pregnancy/ Paediatrics

1998	PB	312pp	38 line illus	ISBN 0 340 74085 X	£35.00